Language Intervention with School-Aged Children
Conversation, Narrative, and Text

Language Intervention with School-Aged Children
Conversation, Narrative, and Text

Rita C. Naremore, Ph.D.

Professor
Indiana University
Bloomington, Indiana

with

Ann E. Densmore, M.A.

Clinical Associate Professor
Indiana University
Bloomington, Indiana

Deborah R. Harman, M.A.T.

Speech-Language Pathologist
Brown County School Corporation
Nashville, Indiana

SINGULAR PUBLISHING GROUP, INC.
San Diego · London

Published by Singular Publishing Group, Inc.
401 West "A" Street, Suite 325
San Diego, California 92101

19 Compton Terrace
London N1 2UN, U.K.

e-mail: singpub@mail.cerfnet.com
Website: http://www.singpub.com

©1995 by Singular Publishing Group, Inc.

Reprinted February 1997
Reprinted November 1997

Typeset in 10/12 Trump Medieval by So Cal Graphics
Printed in the United States of America by McNaughton & Gunn

Library of Congress Cataloging-in-Publication Data

Naremore, Rita C.
    Language intervention with school-aged children : conversation,
    narrative, and text / Rita C. Naremore with Ann E. Densmore and
    Deborah R. Harman.
        p. cm.
    Includes bibliographical references (p.) and index.
    ISBN 1-56593-222-6
    1. Children—Language—Case studies. 2. Language disorders in
    children—Case studies. 3. Communicative competence in children—
    Study and teaching. I. Densmore, Ann E. II. Harman, Deborah R.
    III. Title.
LB1139.L3N29 1994
371.91'4—dc20   94-27442
                                                              CIP

CONTENTS

CHAPTER 9

ACKNOWLEDGEMENTS

No book like this could possibly have appeared in print without the contributions, both witting and unwitting, of many people. We wish to thank them now.

First, we thank the students in our classes in school age language, who learned along with us, and whose creative thinking kept us excited about the possibilities for change.

Next, we thank the colleagues who listened to us, who gave us their reactions, and who encouraged us throughout the writing of this book. Their cheerful inquiries about "how's it going" and their never-faltering belief in us were a great help.

We are grateful as well to Bob Harman and David Fenske, who endured our late nights and weekends of work, and who served as unpaid computer consultants. We promise them a couple of decent meals, now that the work is done.

Ron Gillam, who read the manuscript when it was in an earlier incarnation, deserves our thanks as well. His insightful comments helped us make this a better book. Many of the good things, including Chapter 9, we did at his instigation.

Finally, we wish to dedicate this book to the children, the clinicians, the teachers, and the parents whose lives we have excerpted in our case studies. Their struggles and triumphs served as our learning laboratories, and provided us with the content for this book.

For all of those we have mentioned, and for others who, although they were not mentioned by name, played roles in the generation of this text, THANK YOU!

PREFACE

This book is intended for speech-language pathologists who are working or will be working with language impaired children in school settings. Our goal is to help you feel confident about working with children whose language problems result from difficulties with *higher level language processes*. When we talk about higher level language processes, we are referring to those processes which are necessary for creating and understanding language beyond the sentence level—that language we call "paragraphs" or "stories" or "explanations," to use just a few of the terms we employ for extended prose. Some of the processes involved include the ability to communicate ideas via language alone, without contextual cues; the ability to linguistically represent mental scripts of events; the ability to create cohesive narratives by using specific linguistic devices; the ability to decide how much or how little information a listener needs, etc. We refer to these abilities, and others we will discuss in the book, as "language processes" because they are all important abilities for those **language acts** we call **conversation, narration, and comprehension and creation of text**. It is precisely these three language acts we will address in this book, because, in our experience, they are language acts which are extremely difficult for school-aged language impaired children. Not only that, they are also language acts which are critical to the child's social and academic success in the school environment. Our primary concern as clinical professionals must surely be to maximize the child's chances for succeeding in the day-to-day environment. For the school-aged child, that day-to-day environment is the classroom and the peer group. If a child can't carry on a conversation, if narrative structure is nonexistent, and if it is impossible to fall back on linguistic textual conventions to understand what you read and organize what you write, then the chances for success in the classroom and the peer group are minimal.

Our belief about the cause of these important problems for the school-aged child influences our clinical approach to language impairment in the school-aged population. Specifically, as you will find in Chapter 1, we advocate an environmentally based approach to deciding who is language impaired. Essentially, a child whose language abilities prevent effective functioning in the classroom or the peer group is, by our definition, language impaired. The trick, of course, is to decide which of the children who are rejected by their peer groups or who are failing in school are having these problems as a result of language difficulties, as opposed to cognitive disorders or physical limitations, or other sorts of handicaps. In Chapter 1, we will begin a series of **clinical brainstorming sessions** in which the three of us will allow you to listen in as we discuss **case studies** presented in the text. These sessions will lead to **assessment strategies**, which we will describe for you in further elaborations of the case studies. At the conclusion of Chapter 1, you should have a sense of how we decide which children are having language problems affecting their social or educational success.

We will address the three language acts which are our focus in a particular intervention context, which we will lay out for you in some detail. Specifically, we believe strongly that both the children we're trying to help and we as clinicians will benefit from working in a **collaborative, classroom based context**. We will explain what we mean by these terms, and give you some concrete examples in the second chapter of the book. We will follow up on the case studies presented in Chapter 1, to illustrate how intervention with our two example children might be approached in a collaborative, classroom based model. Then, in the specific intervention chapters, when we talk about children who have problems with conversation, or narrative, or text, our suggestions will all derive from the principles we establish in Chapter 2.

Following these two beginning chapters, in which we will lay the groundwork and establish the principles for further discussions, we will consider each of the three key language acts in turn. Chapter 3 will discuss **conversation**, and the kinds of problems language impaired school-aged children are likely to have with conversation. A detailed case study of a child whose primary language problem appeared in conversation will be presented. Then, in Chapter 4, we will make suggestions for goals and objectives, giving extended examples of intervention activities.

Chapter 5 will focus on **narrative**, and we'll talk about what school-aged children should be able to do with scripts and stories, and present some approaches to assessment. In Chapter 6, we will present several case studies of children having trouble with narratives, along with statements of goals and objectives and extended examples of intervention activities both in and out of the classroom. The last pair of chapters, 7 and 8, will deal with the child's encounter with text. We will discuss why text is different from any of the kinds of language the child has encountered previously, and we will lay out some of the kinds of problems language impaired children have with text in Chapter 7. Chapter 8 will contain goals and objectives for a child introduced in a case study in Chapter 7, and will present extended examples of intervention activities in and out of the classroom.

Then in a final chapter, we present a reprise of the philosophy which guides us as we think and write about school practice.

Throughout the book, you will find helps for you as a reader. Key terms will be defined in blocks. Relevant research literature will be summarized in the text. In Appendixes to the book, you will find a description of all the assessment tools we mention in the text, both commercially available and informal, as well as examples of forms and report formats likely to be found in the cumulative files of language impaired children in the schools.

CHAPTER 1

Identifying the School-Aged Child Who Is Language Impaired

Marilyn S., a school speech-language pathologist in a midwestern school district, was looking over the referrals for her annual beginning of the year assessments. She took particular note of four of the 21 children who had been referred by teachers:

Mitch was a first grader who had been classified language impaired as a preschooler. He was a slow language learner, and had been held out of kindergarten for a year while he continued to receive language intervention at a local clinic. His first grade teacher had asked for a complete psycho-educational assessment because, as a kindergartener, Mitch had made no progress with phonics and seemed to be having difficulty following directions in class. In addition, the kindergarten teacher reported that he was extremely reticent, even with the other children.

Montez was an African-American child whose first grade teacher reported that she couldn't understand much of what he said in class. She gave several examples of his utterances, including "I ain't wear no shirt like that" and "You got teacher pencil in your pocket" and "What kind of work we do in school today?" The teacher's report cited "many errors involving verb usage" combined with "frequent sound errors such as 'teef' for 'teeth'; 'tes' for 'test'; 'bruver' for 'brother'; and 'dis' for 'this'."

Jackie was a third grader who was referred by the learning disabilities resource teacher, who suspected a language problem. Jackie had transferred in from another school system where she had been classified as learning disabled. Jackie was reading at a first grade level, and her teachers reported that she had difficulty with concepts associated with time, measurement, and money. The problems which caused the resource teacher to ask for an assessment, however, were her difficulty following directions in the classroom and her frequent episodes of "getting lost in the middle of her talking, as though she forgot what she was trying to say."

Anna was also a recent transfer into the school system. She was the youngest child of a migrant family who had moved into the area to help with agricultural harvests and had stayed due to the illness of the mother. Anna was eight years old, but had apparently had only one year of school. The family had moved around so much that it was impossible to find a complete school record anywhere. The parents both spoke Spanish in the home, although the father spoke reasonable English. The mother's English was limited to very short utterances, primarily questions such as "Where is doctor?" and "What you want?" She did appear to understand most of what was said to her if the speaker remembered to speak slowly and clearly. Anna's English was much like her mother's. She spoke Spanish at home, and used English only in the classroom. The teacher reported that in the three weeks school had been in session, her vocabulary had grown rapidly, but she was concerned that Anna was not learning English grammar.

Marilyn would have to assess each of these children to discover whether any of them should be called language impaired, and she would need to consult with other professionals who were involved in the assessments about the best placement for each child, and what kinds of services each should receive. Her task was not unlike that faced by many school speech-language professionals at the beginning of an academic year.

WHO SHOULD BE CALLED LANGUAGE IMPAIRED?

The four cases Marilyn had to deal with seem quite different on the surface. However, two of these chidren were eventually classified as language impaired. To understand how one label could apply to children so different from one another, we need to look for the underlying similarities in their cases, and in the cases of all those other children who fit within this classification. What does it mean to say that a school-aged child is language impaired? What is the difference between being language impaired and being learning disabled or mildly mentally handicapped, or just academically below average?

Throughout this book, our approach to language impairment will be grounded in what the child is able to do with language. Our answer to the first question asked above is: **a school aged language impaired child is one who cannot use language to meet the demands of the social and/or academic contexts of the school.** Children who are language impaired are likely to be in trouble academically. They will have trouble learning to read, they will not be good writers, and they will have difficulty learning any subject material which is presented to them through language rather than through, say, concrete demonstration. These are children who, as preschoolers, may have had trouble learning language, and as school aged children they will have difficulty using language to learn.

When we confront the issue of how to discriminate language impaired children from other children who may be having problems in school, we must first recognize the fact that labels do not always describe children's problems very well. A child may be learning disabled **and** language impaired. A child may be mentally handicapped **and** language impaired. Wearing some other label does not mean that the child's language skills are normal. In fact, as we observe over and over again, language impaired children are often relabeled when they start to school, so the child who was labeled language impaired as a preschooler may be called learning disabled or reading disabled or even autistic as an elementary schooler (Bashir, Kuban, Kleinman, & Scavuzzo, 1983; Snyder, 1984; Wallach & Liebergott, 1984). Part of the difficulty here, as Bashir (1986) and others (Fowler, 1986, Spreen & Haaf, 1986) make clear, is that language impairment changes over time. The preschool child who is having difficulty mastering verb morphology may become the third grader whose verb forms sound fine but who cannot summarize a paragraph in the Social Studies textbook. As Wallach and Miller (1988) point out, "Many children in learning disability (LD) and reading classes have ongoing problems with language. The challenge to us in the schools is to learn more about the interactions among children's learning styles, their inherent language abilities, the curricula they are exposed to, and their classroom environments" (p. 5).

This is no small challenge. How do we begin to answer it? Perhaps the simplest way is to take a look first at the child's academic and social progress. Is the child making general academic progress at a rate that is acceptable to teachers and parents? Is the child passing school subjects? Does the child have friends? Is the child able to function on the playground and in the social milieu of a peer group? If the answer to these questions is yes, then we don't need to go further in assessing the child. The child's language abilities, whatever they are, are sufficient to allow functioning in the environment. But what if the answer to these questions is no? What if the child is failing or experiencing major academic difficulty in school, or is unable to find a place in the peer group? Then we need to take a closer look, to determine whether difficulties with language might be contributing to the problem. By thinking about the child's language in light of the child's ability to function in the communication environment, we are advocating a change in the approach many clinicians take to language impairment. In effect, we are saying that we should not depend on a test score, or even a series of test scores, as the only way to tell whether a child is language impaired. Testing can tell us something about the child's strengths and weaknesses, or about the child's knowledge of particular language structures. But only observation of the child in the classroom and playground environments can tell us whether the child can handle the language demands of the environment.

This may sound like ordinary common sense to those not familiar with the current controversy over the definition of "specific language impairment." However, those who are or will be working within the bounds of the sorts of criteria some state education agencies have laid down for deciding who is language impaired will recognize the unusual nature of this statement. For example, Nye and Montgomery (1989) conducted a survey of state education agencies to determine what criteria they were using to identify language impairment. They report that at least 16 states required the use of standardized tests and discrepancy formulas in the identification of language impaired children. That is, these states required clinicians to use standardized tests and identify a significant discrepancy between a child's language test scores and IQ or school achievement scores. Or, the district might require the clinician to demonstrate a difference between the child's language test scores and the scores of other children in his or her age group, or at his or her IQ level. However, there was little agreement from state to state about what constituted a "significant discrepancy," and also about what to compare the child's language test scores to in order to find a discrepancy. In spite of this general lack of agreement, school systems and researchers alike continue to try to come up with test-based definitions of language impairment. Since we cannot ignore the existence of these attempts, we will explain why we consider them both misguided and doomed to failure.

ATTEMPTS TO DEFINE SPECIFIC LANGUAGE IMPAIRMENT

First, it is important to be aware that most of the definitional controversy in this area surrounds the term "specific language impairment," which is generally taken to refer to language impairment without any known cause. Known causes of language impairment include such conditions as hearing impairment, traumatic brain injury, mental retardation, and other impairments of neurological or cognitive functioning. There is little controversy about the fact that children with these conditions have problems with language, and to a degree, we can predict what kinds of language problems they will have. However, it is more difficult to agree about the nature of the problems presented by those children who appear to be having difficulty learning or using language, but for whom no causal factors can be identified. It is this "specific language impairment," as opposed to "language impairment secondary to hearing loss" or "language impairment secondary to traumatic brain injury" that we have so much trouble defining.

As Aram, Morris, and Hall (1993) point out, typical definitions of language impairment have included the use of both discrepancy and exclusionary criteria. **Exclusionary criteria are used to differentiate those children with specific language impairments not attributable to known causes from children whose language or learning impairments may be attributed to known factors, such as mental retardation or hearing impairment.** Exclusionary criteria, then, are provided to help eliminate certain children from the category we label "specific language impaired." **Discrepancy criteria, on the other hand, involve identifying a disparity between the impaired function, such as language, and some other nonimpaired aspect of cognitive functioning.** The primary reason for having discrepancy criteria in a definition of language impairment is to show that the child's language ability is significantly below what might be expected based on the child's age or intelligence. For example, a child may demonstrate a discrepancy between language abilities (as indicated by the calculation of "language age" based on a score on a test) and grade level or chronological age; or, a child might score significantly lower on some language test than other children of the same age. A discrepancy based definition of specific language impairment might say something like: *The child must demonstrate a severe discrepancy (at least 1.5 s.d.) between performance on a standardized test of language development and the average performance of children of the same chronological age. This discrepancy may occur in all, one, or some combination of the phonological, semantic, and syntactic components of language, and may be manifested in either comprehension, production or both.* This definition, in common with other discrepancy based definitions, tells us first how much discrepancy we should look for (1.5 standard deviations below the mean) and what we are comparing the child's language to (that of other children the same age).

> The *standard deviation* of a set of test scores is a measure of the variance of the scores around the mean. It might be thought of as an average of all the deviations from the mean. In a normally distributed set of scores, 16% of scores will be 1 s.d. above the mean, and 16% of scores will be 1 s.d. below the mean. The set of scores obtained when a test is standardized is always presumed to be normally distributed.

The goal of definitions of language impairment using exclusion criteria and discrepancy statements is to identify children whose problems with language (1) cannot be ascribed to any readily identifiable cause, such as hearing impairment, and (2) are of sufficient magnitude to justify intervention. The assumption seems to be that we don't need a definition to help us decide whether hearing impairment or traumatic brain injury cause language impairment—we know that they do. The focus of our concern with definitions is those children who seem to be having trouble learning language for unknown reasons. When we find such children, we need to be certain that they are not just experiencing some temporary delay in the process of language acquisition. In other words, if the child's language problems are not significantly below what we would expect based on the child's chronological or mental age, then we should leave the child alone and wait for him or her to catch up. In short, these sorts of criteria are designed to help us decide who needs clinical intervention for language problems. Logical and neat as this sounds, such definitions are not without problems. There is general agreement about exclusion criteria based on known causes of language impairment, but the discrepancy part of the definition has created many sources of confusion.

CONFUSIONS CREATED BY TEST-BASED DEFINITIONS

There are two problems associated with test-based definitions of language impairment. First, using tests to determine who is language impaired must be based on the assumption that tests measure what we need to know about the child's language ability. We believe that standardized language tests are poor measures of what children actually know about language. First, a test by its nature samples only a small subset of the behaviors we include under the label "language." Most of them focus on vocabulary, morphology, and syntax. Very few examine the kinds of higher level language processes needed to understand stories and paragraphs, or the sorts of language processes needed to compose and express extended discourse such as event recounting or story telling—language processes involved in organizing information, deciding how much or how little a listener needs to know, or expanding descriptions. The typical assessment focus on syntax and morphology is probably not useful for identifying many school aged children who are language impaired, since their problems tend to surface in other ways. As Lahey (1990) points out, "procedures for identifying children with language disorders [should] include tasks that stress the use of the language system so that difficulties in performance would most likely be evident" (p. 55). In addition, although we have little information about how language impaired children change over time, we know that they do develop language. A child whose syntactic abilities at age 4 years may be well below those of other children his age will develop syntax. By the time this child is 10 years old, his syntax may not be that far below normal, but his ability to provide an extended description of a science experiment may be far below that of other children his age. The first problem with discrepancy based definitions, in other words, is that we don't know whether the discrepancy stays the same over time, and tests don't give us a very good picture of what we want to measure to find the discrepancy in the first place.

Second, a testing situation is an artificial setting which does not call for functional language use in the service of communication, and does not provide the child with normal contextual support for language use. Children are prevented from using their full knowledge of language in a test situation. Any practicing clinician who has done much language testing will tell you stories of children who failed to use past tense morphemes or auxiliary verbs in a testing situation, and then were heard to use them in a discussion in the classroom, or when recounting an experience. Testing situations represent the most "decontextualized" settings any child is ever likely to encounter. Because of this, language tests force children to think and talk about language rather than using it as a tool to convey their ideas and feelings. This metalinguistic focus in the testing situation is equivalent to asking a carpenter to think and talk about a hammer instead of demonstrating its use.

Metalinguistic awareness enables us to hold language as an object of perception—to think about, talk about and analyze language form separately from meaning. When we count the number of words in a sentence, or when we listen to a sentence to decide whether it is grammatical, we are using our metalinguistic abilities. When children first learn language,

(continued)

(continued)

they learn it as a tool to use for communicating meaning, and metalinguistic awareness develops later. Chapter 7 contains a more extended discussion of metalinguistic awareness.

Difficulties of this sort in the testing situation confound the interpretation of language test scores, and raise reasonable doubts about whether a test score should be taken as an indication of a child's language knowledge or ability to use language in everyday life. We have taken an approach to language impairment which demands that we attend to the child's use of language in the ordinary communication environment, and we prefer to use tests only to answer specific questions about specific areas of language performance, such as following directions or comprehending text.

Another serious source of confusion resulting from test-based discrepancy definitions revolves around the fact that they encourage dependence on tests by implying that tests provide an objective measure of a child's language knowledge that is both more reliable and more valid than a clinician's informed observation of a child's language use. In fact, if a clinician's goal is to decide whether a given child is language impaired, using a score on a standardized language test as the basis for the decision is among the worst procedures.

As Fazio, Naremore, and Connell (1993) point out, the basic reason why a low score on a standardized test of language development cannot be equated with displaying the symptoms of language impairment has to do with the fact that while a child either does or does not have a language impairment (a dichotomous scale), test scores may vary along a continuous scale (from 0 to 100). If we want to use test scores to define language impairment, we must impose the dichotomous either/or scale over the continuous test score scale. In other words, somewhere between 0 and 100 on the test, we have to draw a line and say that anyone scoring below that line is language impaired, and anyone scoring above it is not. The place where we draw that line is entirely arbitrary. The fact that we are using a number (a test score) to define language impairment does not mean we are being objective. The test does not provide us with any information about what score indicates impairment. Our decision about how low a score has to be to indicate a language impairment must be made on a purely *subjective* rather than objective basis. There is no magic test score that always indicates language impairment. In fact, the situation we face with scores on standardized language tests is quite the opposite. *All our available standardized language tests were standardized using only children known to have normal language. Any child believed to have a language impairment was excluded from the standardization group.* This means that when you look at the range of scores in any test manual, and set your cut-off line for defining language impairment, *some percentage of the normal children who took the test (and, presumably, any other normal children who take it) will have scores below that line.* If you find the mean score for 6-year-old children, and decide that any 6 year old who scores more than 1 standard deviation below that mean on the test will be called language impaired, you must recognize that 16% of the normal 6 year olds who took it for standardization purposes scored 1 standard deviation below the mean. This fact is a function of the statistical model used in test standardization. In short, if you use standardized test scores to define language impairment, you will be defining language impairment purely in terms of normal children's test performance. An analogy might be drawn between our task and that of a physician diagnosing measles. There is a clear line between those who have measles and those who do not. We can only tell who has measles by observing the symptoms of the disease and determining whether a child does or does not have them. On the other hand, the model used by most language development tests assumes that the normality line can be drawn without reference to the performance of abnormal language users. That is, test makers standardize these tests on groups composed only of normally developing children who have no sign of language problems. Using the test scores of children who are known to be normal language users to decide who is language impaired is like looking at a group of well children to decide who has measles. No matter where we decide to draw the line on the continuum of test scores to designate language impairment, some of the children who score below the line are certain to be normal.

If we don't use a standard deviation cut-off for deciding who is language impaired, then what about using age equivalency scores? This method also presents us with an unavoidable overlap between scores of children known to be normal and those labeled language impaired. Suppose that Johnny, who is exactly 7 years old, receives age equivalent scores on the *Test of Language Development 2-Primary* (TOLD-2P; Newcomer & Hammill, 1988) that meet the frequently used criteria for language impairment of Stark and Tallal (1981). [Note: This test, and all other assessment instruments or methods mentioned in the book, are described in Appendix 2.] These criteria first exclude children with hearing, emotional, cognitive, neurological, or severe speech impairments, and then define the necessary test score discrepancies as:

1. at least a one-year difference between CA (or MA, whichever is lower) and expressive language age score
2. at least a six-month difference between CA (or MA) and receptive language age score
3. at least a 12-month difference between CA (or MA) and a composite language age score

Specifically, let's say that Johnny receives a Listening Quotient score of 93, which translates into a receptive age equivalent score of 6:6, showing a 6 month delay; a Speaking Quotient of 86, which translates into an expressive age equivalent score of 6:0, showing a 12 month delay, and a Spoken Language Quotient of 86 which translates to a composite age equivalent score of 6:0, or a 12 month delay. He also receives a score on a test of nonverbal intelligence of 90, which is within one standard deviation of the mean. Since only normal children were used to standardize the test, by looking at the score distribution, we can predict that 25% of normal-language 7-year-olds would have the same or lower receptive age score as Johnny, 16% would have the same or lower expressive age score, and 16% would have the same or lower composite age equivalent score. This blurring of normal and abnormal is the direct result of attempting to define what is abnormal (specific language impairment) by reference only to what is normal (scores of the standardization group on the test).

Some people have responded that the way to deal with these facts is to set the cutoff for language impairment further from the mean on our standardized language tests. This would certainly result in fewer normal children being misidentified as language impaired, but it would lead to two other problems: first, a more stringent criterion might fail to identify some children who are truly language impaired but who do not score poorly enough on the test to meet the cutoff criterion. This possibility relates to questions about the *validity* of tests like the TOLD-2P as measures of language development, which will be discussed shortly. Second, re-setting the cutoff point would not eliminate the basic problem, because normal children have scores across the entire distribution of scores on the test. The flaw in the logic of the standardized test approach to identifying language impairment is not a matter of where we draw the line between normal and impaired. The flaw is that wherever the line is drawn, it will be placed somewhere within the distribution of scores that normal children receive, since that is what the continuum of scores is composed of. Moving the cutoff point closer to the lower end of the distribution of scores only makes sense if there is a second group of subjects to move towards. Otherwise, the overlap between normal and abnormal will continue to exist. In other words, normality has to be defined with reference to two groups of children—both those who are normal language learners and those who are not.

The question of the validity of standardized language tests like the TOLD-2P was raised earlier in regard to whether we should move the cutoff for language impairment closer to the lower extreme of the normal distribution. Test validity refers to our assurance that the test measures what we think it is measuring. It is a complex issue which has been discussed often in our literature (McCauley & Swisher, 1984; Stephens & Montgomery, 1985). Everyone is uncomfortable with the practice of saying that a given language test is valid because it correlates highly with other language tests. The fact that two tests are measuring the same thing does not necessarily mean that either of them is measuring a child's language ability. There is no ultimate criterion for deciding how valid tests of language development actually are, and this is at the heart of the entire controversy about definitions of language impairment.

After this lengthy discussion of what is wrong with test-based definitions, it is reasonable to ask why anyone would attempt to define language impairment in terms of test scores. Part of the explanation involves our need for some common, standard definition about which clinicians and researchers might agree. Having a single definition of specific language impairment that could be applied in every setting, whether clinical or research, would be of great benefit to us. With such a definition, we would all know exactly what was meant when a clinical report or a research article mentioned that a child was language impaired. Unfortunately, this may be an unrealistic goal. Meeting this goal would require us to have standardized tests of language much more valid and reliable than any test we have available now. It would also imply that language impaired children are the same across time; that is, that the discrepancy between age-level expectations and the child's performance on the test remained the same for a 7-year-old as for a 4-year-old. In addition, test based definitions seem to imply that there is one profile of scores that would adequately describe all children who have language impairments, or that there is only one kind of language impaired child. None of the research about language impairment published to date suggests that any of this is the case.

Many of the problems with the discrepancy approach to defining specific language impairment have been recognized by the American Speech-Language-Hearing Association (1989). Specifically, ASHA's concern was with the practice of basing decisions about eligibility for language intervention on discrepancy formulas such as those adopted by many state educational agencies. Several problems with discrepancy definitions were addressed in the ASHA report, including:

1. the use of a single aspect of language, such as expressive syntax, in determining a discrepancy;
2. the lack of available valid, technically adequate age-appropriate instruments;
3. the creation of a false sense of objectivity and precision among diagnosticians backed by "statistically based" decisions;
4. reduction in the number of individuals served;
5. failure to provide important qualitative information regarding the nature of the language or learning deficits;
6. the psychometrically incorrect practice of comparing test scores derived from differing theoretical bases and standardization populations.

As the report says, "The exclusive use of a discrepancy formula as a required procedure for determining eligibility for language intervention should be viewed with extreme caution and avoided whenever possible" (ASHA, 1989, p. 115).

TEST SCORES AND CLINICAL JUDGMENT

Further evidence for the inadequacy of discrepancy definitions can be found in the work of Aram, Morris, and Hall (1993), who are concerned with the fact that children identified as language impaired by clinicians are often not the same ones who would be identified by the strict application of a test-based discrepancy criterion. These researchers identified 252 children between the ages of three and five who had been diagnosed as language impaired by clinicians in one of five sites in the eastern US. They then tested each child individually using the *Stanford-Binet Intelligence Scale—Revised* (Thorndyke, Hagen, & Sattler, 1986) and the *Test of Early Language Development* (TELD; Hresko, Reid, & Hammill, 1981). The Stanford Binet was used to obtain IQ measures, and the TELD to obtain a quantitative measure of overall language functioning. Various other language measures were used, including MLU taken from a spontaneous language sample, and the standard score from the Communication Domain of the *Vineland Adaptive Behavior Scales* (Sparrow, Balla, & Cicchetti, 1984) completed through an interview with the child's parent or primary caregiver. The authors summarize their results as follows:

A review of these results revealed the greatest congruence between clinical judgment and research identification of SLI in children was achieved using one of the following criteria: the Stanford-Binet-TELD discrepancy criterion of equal to or greater than one standard deviation [identified 59.1%], the Stanford-Binet-Vineland Communication Domain discrepancy of one standard deviation or greater [identified 60%], or the criterion of an MLU standard age score below 85 [identified 71.4%]. While the Vineland appears to have usefulness in identifying children with SLI, it is not often reported in research in SLI nor is it always available clinically. Thus, in applying both the Stanford-Binet-TELD and MLU cut-off criteria (which are more widely recognized clinically and in research), 201 of the original 252 clinically defined children (79.8%) were identified as SLI. (p. 585)

In discussing these results, the authors point out that "one should not expect any one test, or clinical procedure to have stable sensitivity and specificity for a particular diagnostic decision across the developmental spectrum or range of populations with different base-rates of SLI" (p. 588).

The results of this study are echoed in a longitudinal study conducted by Fazio et al. (1993). These researchers followed three groups of children from kindergarten through second grade. One group of children was identified as being at risk for language impairment as kindergarteners, based on their performance on the TOLD-2P. To be placed in the at-risk group, a child had to have a nonverbal IQ (measured by the *Columbia Mental Maturity Scale* (CMMS) of 85 or above and at least two subtest scores on the TOLD-2P at one standard deviation or greater below the mean. A second group of children with normal TOLD-2P scores was matched with this group on the basis of nonverbal IQ and classroom. A third group of children, identified as slow developers, had nonverbal IQ scores of less than 85 and TOLD-2P scores like those of the children in the at-risk group. In addition to the TOLD-2P and the CMMS, these researchers also administered several non-traditional language measures, in an attempt to derive some set of measures which could be used to predict which children might be language impaired at the end of first grade. As a part of their data analysis, Fazio et al. applied Stark and Tallal's discrepancy definition, using the children's scores on the TOLD-2P in kindergarten, first, and second grades. The Stark and Tallal criterion identified nine children as SLI based on kindergarten scores—eight from the at risk group and one from the group identified as normal by Fazio et al. At the end of first grade, use of the Stark and Tallal criterion identified nine children again, six of whom had been identified at the end of kindergarten and three of whom had not. Of these nine children, only three had been identified by school speech-language pathologists and were receiving services. In other words, Fazio et al. found the same lack of overlap between children identified using a discrepancy definition and children identified by practicing clinicians as Aram et al. had found. Interestingly, while Aram et al. found that the discrepancy approach underidentified language impaired children, the Fazio et al. study found that it overidentified. Part of this apparent contradiction may be due to the different ages of the children involved in the two studies.

As we mentioned above, one of the goals of the Fazio et al. study was to derive a set of measures that might present a better match with clinical definitions of SLI. These researchers developed three independent measures: a story retelling task, a morpheme learning task, and a rote memory task, which they administered to the children at each grade level. The authors set a cut-off criterion which would eliminate any overlap between children classified as language impaired and children known in advance to be normal. Using this criterion (failure on two out of three of the tasks), seven children were identified as SLI at the end of first grade. Five of the seven had also been identified independently by the school speech-language pathologists. These findings suggest that objective measurement criteria and clinical judgment are not necessarily incompatible, but discrepancy criteria do not provide the sort of compatibility we might hope for.

A CLINICAL APPROACH FOR PRACTICAL PURPOSES

This wide circle brings us back to the original question: what are we supposed to look at, as clinicians, to decide which children are language impaired and in need of services? Our answer to that question may sound less objective than the discrepancy based definitions quoted earlier in this chapter, but this characteristic is outweighed by its utility in the school setting.

Our clinical approach to identifying a school-aged language impaired child is to focus on **any child who is unable to use language to meet the demands of the communication environment.** For the school-aged child, the relevant communication environment is the classroom and the age-matched peer group. From this definition, we derive our identification strategies.

First, FOCUS on the child in the language environment. Take a look at how the child is functioning in the school classroom and on the playground. Is the child experiencing significant academic difficulty? Is the child struggling with literacy? Has the child been held back in school? Is the child experiencing significant social problems, such as inability to make friends or rejection by other children in his or her age group? If the answer is yes, proceed.

Second, OBSERVE. Take a look at the child's language use across a variety of situations. Listen to what the teacher says about the child. Observe the child in the classroom and on the playground. Does the child comprehend the teacher's instructions in the classroom? Can the child use language to get clarification when misunderstandings occur? Can the child carry on a conversation with the teacher? Can the child participate in group discussions in the classroom? Can the child use language to recount events and to tell and respond to stories? Can the child participate in routine playground activities with other children? Can the child enter an already constituted group of peers and be accepted as a participant? How does the child's language use compare with that of other children in the classroom or on the playground?

Third, instead of focusing on which standardized test you might give, **THINK** about what the classroom is demanding of the child. Teachers and textbooks make certain assumptions about what children come to school knowing. Does this child know what we assume he or she knows about language? How are the child's metalinguistic abilities? What does the child know about narrative structure? Can this child introduce a new topic in a conversation, and shift topics smoothly? Can the child use textbooks and other material provided in the classroom to learn new material? Can the child find the important information in a paragraph of text, and use this information to answer questions about the paragraph? In answering these questions, it will be necessary for you to do some nontraditional testing, using story retelling, for example, or adapting methods used in the research literature for assessment purposes. The use of clinician constructed or informal testing may require you to develop local norms for some of the tests you use frequently. How to do this will be described in case study discussion throughout the book.

Finally, DO SOME SPECIFIC TESTING. Zero in on some of those areas of language use where the child appears to be having trouble, and do some in-depth exploration. Use commercially available tests where they are likely to help. If you believe that lack of ability to use syntax or morphology is the source of a child's problems, then test for the child's understanding and production of syntax and morphology. **But do not stop there.** For example, if a teacher reports that a child does not follow directions well in class, you might administer the Oral Directions or the

Linguistic Concepts subtests of the *Clinical Evaluation of Language Fundamentals—Revised* (CELF-R; Semel, Wiig, & Secord, 1987) to help you find out more about the problem. If the child is having problems comprehending what she reads, you might start with the paragraph comprehension subtest on the CELF-R, and check also on inferencing abilities by adapting some of the measures used in the research literature (see Chapter 7 for further discussion of inferencing). One word of caution is in order here: when you administer only certain subtests of a commercially available test, you should not then use the test norms as the basis for deciding whether the child is language impaired. Your goal here is to get a closer look at specific areas of language use, not to attempt to derive a "language age" or something of that sort. In addition, as we pointed out in step three, commercially available tests need not be your only source for probing specific areas of a child's language performance. In many cases, you may want to examine language processes not covered by such tests. In these cases, you should not be afraid to develop your own measures, based on what researchers have done. You may even administer these tasks to children you know to be language-normal and to children you know to be language impaired, to get a feel for how their performance differs.

WHO IS DEFINITELY NOT LANGUAGE IMPAIRED?

Any definition of language impairment, or any approach to identifying language impaired children, should exclude children who are normal speakers of social or ethnic dialects, or who are learning English as a second language. Children learn the language of their environments. If the child's parents speak Spanish, the child will learn Spanish. If the child's parents speak a regional dialect, such as the familiar Southern or Boston or New York dialects, so will the child. If the child's parents speak an ethnic dialect, such as the one used by many African-American people in America, the child will speak this dialect. If the child's language is like that spoken by the parents, the child is not language impaired. There is no dialect of English which would cause a child to experience significant academic difficulties. Certainly, dialect speakers can suffer social consequences in some environments. Children may tease others who sound "funny," and American society penalizes dialect speakers in some social or occupational environments. This does not mean, however, that the dialect speaker is language impaired. The great majority of children using social or ethnic dialects are perfectly normal, just as are the great majority of children speaking more mainstream varieties of English. The challenge to the clinician is to separate out the influence of a dialect from the influence of a language impairment. This is a situation in which comparing a child with other speakers of the dialect will be useful, as will more in-depth objective testing to discover how the child uses language in particular contexts. What will most assuredly not be useful will be administering tests of syntax or morphology which were designed for and standardized on speakers of a dialect other than that used by the child.

This discussion is particularly relevant if the child in question is a speaker of English as a second language. One of the biggest changes in school practice over the last decade has been the increasing numbers of children in the schools for whom English is not the first language. Many of these children will learn English, perhaps with instruction, perhaps just as a result of being in an English-speaking environment. Some of them, however, will experience academic problems and will have great difficulty with the second language learning process. Deciding when a second-language learner has a language impairment is a challenge for any clinician, if only because the best way to determine this is to test the child in his or her native language, and that demands an adult speaker of that language who understands the diagnostic enterprise. We should also increase our search for culture free tests of children's language learning ability, such as the one used by Roseberry and Connell (1991) to identify language impaired Spanish speaking children. Several books are already available to provide help for clinicians working with multicultural populations, and more are undoubtedly on the way. It is not our intention here to cover this understandably troublesome area of clinical practice. We have only two points to make: a dialect, or English influenced by some other language having been learned first, is not a language impairment. Speakers of dialects or of English as a second language may be language impaired, however, and assessing these children demands great care and creativity.

A FINAL WORD ABOUT DECIDING WHO IS LANGUAGE IMPAIRED

School speech-language pathologists must work within the confines of the rules governing practice in their particular states. If you work in a state which requires you to use discrepancy based definitions for deciding who should be in your caseload, you have little choice but to abide by this requirement. This does not mean, however, that you are prevented from employing the approach we have outlined in this chapter. Use our approach to find the children you believe to be language impaired, and then support your findings with discrepancy based testing. In those cases where you believe a child is language impaired, but discrepancy based testing does not support this belief, we suggest that you continue to observe, and continue to test. Work with others in the school, including resource teachers and other special education professionals, to find ways to help the child. No definition and no approach, including ours, should prevent you from finding a way to help a child whose language difficulties are serious enough to result in academic or social failure.

A CLINICAL APPLICATION

Having discussed the issues involved in deciding which children need services from the school speech-language pathologist, let us now return to the four children whose cases we mentioned at the beginning of the chapter. Marilyn S., when she had completed her initial assessments, determined that Montez was a normal speaker of Black English Vernacular (BEV), a dialect spoken by many African-Americans, especially those living in the inner cities of large metropolitan areas. His syntax, morphology, and phonological system were the same as those used by other speakers of the dialect. In her interactions with him, Marilyn discovered that Montez comprehended the mainstream English she spoke, and that he did use mainstream forms occasionally in his own speech. Montez's teacher was unfamiliar with the characteristics of BEV, and had never been around children who spoke the dialect, so Marilyn provided her with some materials about the dialect, and the two of them discussed some ways to help Montez become bi-dialectal in the classroom. Anna presented Marilyn with a more complex problem. She called on the school system's director of special education to locate a native Spanish speaker who could help her evaluate Anna's language ability in her native language. She decided to observe Anna for several weeks to see how her English changed as she interacted with the teacher and the other children in the classroom, and she talked with the teacher about the fact that it might take some time to complete assessment on Anna because of the language differences involved.

Mitch and Jackie, however, presented Marilyn with quite another picture. We will discuss their cases in some detail, because they are representative of the two sorts of children most often seen in school caseloads: children who come into school already classified as language impaired based on problems as preschoolers, and children who are identified as language impaired for the first time after experiencing difficulty in school. Along with our discussion of these children, we have also included copies of their cumulative school records, containing reports from all the professionals who worked with them, and surveys of their academic progress. These folders are located in Appendix 1 of the book, and you may want to refer to them as we discuss the cases below.

MITCH AND JACKIE: EXAMPLES OF LANGUAGE IMPAIRED CHILDREN IN SCHOOL

Case 1. Mitch: The Preschool Language-Impaired Child in the School Setting

Mitch was brought to a university Speech & Hearing Clinic at age three because, according to his parents, he was very slow learning to talk. At the time, his expressive vocabulary was around 50 words, including some social routines such as "hi" and "bye bye," labels for objects, and a few verbs. He was not combining words except in a few routines such as "all gone." His hearing was tested, and found to be normal in both ears. Mitch's score on the *Test of Auditory Comprehension of Language—Revised* (TACL-R; Carrow-Woolfolk, 1985) as well as his performance in interacting with the clinician who conducted the assessment, indicated, however, that his comprehension of language, while lower than might be expected for his age, exceeded his expression. Mitch's father reported that he himself had been a "slow talker," and had experienced great difficulty with reading and writing in school.

Mitch was enrolled in a preschool program for language impaired children, and remained in the program for two years, until he was 5 years old. He showed slow but steady progress, particularly in vocabulary development and in the use of multi-word utterances. At the end of two years, he still had difficulty with the pronouns "I" and "me" (he substituted "me" for "I" frequently) and with the verb "to be." He was able to follow three-step commands, so long as the activities were ones with which he was familiar. He could use language to make his own wants known, and to share his ideas and feelings with others in the environment. In spite of much work, his language skills seemed to desert him in moments of conflict, and he was prone to hit and bite and scream. He also had difficulty retelling experiences, particularly when the context of the experience was not present. He could retell a scripted experience, such as a birthday party held in the classroom, with the aid of pictures. However, he was unable to tell about going to McDonald's, in spite of frequent visits with his family. His attempt to relate this experience was lacking in sequential organization and he tended to focus on minor details rather than on the major events.

Mitch was held out of kindergarten for one year, continuing to receive individual therapy at the clinic. By the time he began kindergarten at age 6 years, his pronoun confusions were over, and verb morphology was usually in place. He was better able to recount scripted events, but was unable to retell even the simplest story, and seemed unable to memorize the simple songs and rhymes taught to him by his clinician. During the year before he began school, his clinicians focused on "school vocabulary" and on some early encounters with print, reading stories to him and printing his own attempts to tell stories as books for him to take home to his family. Most of these books consisted of pictures he had drawn with four or five word descriptive captions. There was little or no narrative structure in any of them.

The next fall, Mitch was enrolled in kindergarten. At the pre-enrollment conference, Mitch's mother brought the Speech & Hearing Center's final report. The kindergarten teacher passed this report on to the speech-language pathologist, and a case conference was scheduled to set goals and objectives for Mitch in kindergarten. It was decided that Mitch would work with the speech-language pathologist twice a week, continuing the kinds of intervention he had been having. In the first weeks of school. the speech-language pathologist observed the interactions between Mitch and the teacher and Mitch and the other children. In discussion with the teacher, the speech-language pathologist shared information about language impairment and the particular language difficulties Mitch might experience. She suggested some classroom adaptations that might help both Mitch and the teacher, such as making sure Mitch was attending before giving him directions. She also retested Mitch's hearing, to make sure it was not a contributing factor, and found it to be normal.

Mitch's kindergarten teacher placed a great deal of emphasis on phonics and learning to print the letters of the alphabet. Mitch experienced difficulty with printing, demonstrating several letter reversals and an apparent inability to stay on the line. His teacher also reported that he was a failure when it came to phonics. She said, "In all my years of teaching I have never had a child who simply was unable to learn the sounds of the letters." She observed that he was a problem in the classroom because he was always asking the other children what he was supposed to be doing. At the year-end case conference, the first grade teacher who would have Mitch the next year was invited to attend. Mitch's individual strengths and weaknesses were discussed. Goals and objectives for the next year were established, and it was decided in conjunction with the parents that the speech-language pathologist and the classroom teacher would closely monitor Mitch's progress, with the idea that he might need a complete psychoeducational assessment.

Following two first grade grading periods in which Mitch continued to struggle with all academic areas, he was referred to the Student Assistance Team. This team evaluates the current program and decides whether further adaptations in the classroom or further testing are needed. The team decided that they would complete a psychoeducational battery, and that they would also conduct a classroom observation and a full communication evaluation.

Mitch was typical in many ways of children who come to school already identified as language impaired. First, his early expressive vocabulary was severely delayed. Second, he had difficulty learning the syntactic and morphological systems of English needed for sentence formulation. Then, even after sentence formulation had apparently been mastered, the higher level language skills needed to encode, organize, and link propositions and to retrieve specific words from storage continued to present problems. Mitch's difficulty with phonics suggests that, as is typical with other children like him, he had not developed the metalinguistic skills needed for sound-letter matching. It is as though his slow start doomed him to be forever behind his peers in developing language skills. Given the extent to which academic instruction depends on such skills, Mitch's failure in the classroom seems inevitable.

Now we are ready to put our clinical approach to the test, and see how it might work in the case of children like Mitch and Jackie. We will illustrate our process by first reporting a clinical brainstorming session, in which we decided what kind of assessment to do, and then we'll give you the results of that assessment. Our purpose in giving you access to our brainstorming about these cases is to present not only the results but also the process involved in clinical decision making. Although we all work with language impaired children, we approach children's language from our individual perspectives and our different experiences. One of the rules of a brainstorming session is that no idea is wrong or inappropriate. A brainstorming session is a time to get everybody's ideas out on the table, before deciding how to proceed. It is a technique that will be very useful in collaboration and group decision making. We do not always agree about what is most important for a given child. Our hope is that, by reading our interactions, you will gain some insight into the kinds of thinking and the kinds of questions that arise when we attempt to assess children's language.

Clinical Brainstorming: Mitch

Before beginning to talk about Mitch, we reviewed what was becoming a rather thick file. (Note: the documents in that file which would be relevant to our discussion are included in Appendix 1. In reality, other documents such as the health record would also be reviewed prior to planning assessment, but we have not included those in Appendix 1, for reasons of space.) We noted the problems he had had as a preschooler, and the results of his kindergarten year. Then, bearing in mind that Mitch was now in first grade, and was a full year older than most of the other children in his class, we began our discussion.

Rita: What strikes you first when you read about this child? What do you want to find out about right off the bat?

Ann: One worrisome piece of data to my mind is this business about following directions. He had so much trouble learning language as a preschooler, and now he's having trouble using language in school. It's as though all his cognitive storage is filled up with just trying to manipulate syntax and morphology, and he doesn't have room for anything else.

Debbie: And yet, his receptive language seems to have been nearly normal when he was a preschooler, at least as far as we could see from the assessment that was done.

Ann: I wonder just how normal that receptive language was. I'm suspicious of that phrase. How much language did he have to know to perform within normal limits on that test at age three?

Debbie: I'm wondering whether he needs more kinds of input. I notice that using pictures helps him to recall a script. Maybe he needs to have everything in a context, to give him something to hang information on.

Ann: Could be. Maybe we should find a script that first graders should know about, like eating lunch in the cafeteria. We could ask him first to order a set of pictures of the event, then ask him to tell us about it. In other words, is he having problems with event representations, even in pictures, or is his problem primarily one of turning these event representations into language?

Rita: I agree with that, but getting back to following directions , I wonder what effect the teacher has. He has a new teacher now, and I'd like to do some observation to find out whether he's still having trouble with this. And, on another topic, I'm probably most worried by this difficulty with phonics, and his failure to learn to read. The report in his folder from the Chapter I reading teacher suggests that he is learning to recognize some words, using a word recognition strategy. Maybe he might actually be able to learn to read if we get away from the decoding problem, but there's no question that he needs some phonics along the line. I'd like to take a look at his metalinguistic abilities. Can he tell how many sounds are in a word? Can he tell what's left if you take off one sound?

The Chapter I program is a federally funded program intended to provide remedial services to children from poverty. The remedial services are generally in reading and math.

Ann: Well, we might as well use the tasks Kamhi and Catts (1986) used in their research as a way of finding out about metalinguistic awareness. And while we're at it, let's test several children in the classroom who the teacher considers "average." That will give us some comparative data, so we'll know whether Mitch really is at a different level in terms of phonological awareness. And I'd like to know why he would be doing better in Chapter I? Smaller class, or different teaching method, or what?

Debbie: Yeah, smaller group. Also, the Chapter I teacher uses a lot of children's literature in her class, and that might give him more context for reading than a basal reader will. If she's focusing on whole word recognition, he might be building up a store of individual content words he can recognize, like "train" or "elephant," while he's still having trouble with function words like "was" and "did." Let's do some observation in that classroom, and see what he does differently, as well as what the teacher does.

Rita: That approach to reading might also enable him to use his world knowledge. He might have an easier time predicting what the word is, because he would know what word would make sense in a given context.

Debbie: I wonder if she's teaching reading around themes? Like a unit on Indians or a unit on animals? If that helps him, it would be a useful thing to know for intervention. That's an important observation to do.

Ann: And how much reading does he get at home? From the sound of it, I'm guessing that's not a household focused on print. I know they worked on stories in therapy when he was a preschooler, but he may need more work on narrative structure. If he doesn't have a story framework, he's going to have trouble with story comprehension, even if he gets past his decoding problems. We've done enough story retelling with normal first graders at this point to have some good data for comparison, so let's have him retell a story for us.

Rita: I'm also concerned about his ability to participate in the classroom. Is he able to carry on a conversation with the teacher? And can he interact appropriately with his peers on the playground? Let's see what we can find out with a conversational analysis. Maybe his language problems are all coming out in the academic setting, and he's actually fine socially.

Ann: Ok, so what are we going to do? We want to look at the following directions problem as well as try to find some explanation for his performance with phonics and in Chapter I reading. So we're going to do some close observation of the classrooms, to find out what the teachers do, and what kinds of difficulties he still seems to be having with classroom discourse, in what contexts. We also want to look at his phonological metalinguistic abilities. [Phonological metalinguistic abilities are described in Chapter 7.] So we'll do some informal testing, using the Kamhi and Catts procedures [these procedures are described in Appendix 3] and we'll test three or four children from his classroom at the same time, to get a fix on what the average child in the room can do with these tasks. And we want to find out about his ability to deal with scripts as long as he's using pictures without words, so we'll do a picture arranging task.

Then we want to see how he does using language, to tell us about a scripted event [scripted event recounting is described in detail in Chapter 5]. Here again, I'd like to get some scripted event recounting from a few average kids in his class, just to have a basis for comparison. And we certainly want to do some story retelling, to find out whether he's catching on to narrative structure [story retelling and narrative structure analysis are described in detail in Chapter 7.] We have some data, built up over time, to tell us how other first grade children do with story retelling, so we can actually use that for comparison purposes. Then, just to get a fix on his social language use, we're going to get a conversation sample and take a look at his conversational appropriacy. [Conversational analysis is described in Chapter 3.] This should keep us busy for a while.

Results of the assessment

We will report the results of this assessment first in terms of what we found from our observations, then what we found from formal and informal testing. Focused observation in the classroom, watching to see how the teacher gave directions and how Mitch coped with them, made it clear that, when the teacher made sure Mitch was paying attention, and when she gave directions slowly, using concrete contexts, such as holding up the page she wanted the children to work on, Mitch was able to do as well as other children in the class. However, when there were other things going on in the room, or when the teacher used complex language and embedded directions in other talk, Mitch failed to catch on. For example, at one point the teacher, sitting with a small group in one corner of the classroom, raised her voice to address the class as a whole, and said, "We have to begin to think about getting to the auditorium for the film we're going to see today. Those of you who have finished your math should start to clear up the paper and paints we left out after art class. And if you're working on your spelling, be sure you get all the words copied off the board before you put your papers away." Several children got up from their seats and began to put away art materials. After looking around for a few minutes, Mitch, who had been copying spelling words, got up and began to help them. Later, the teacher was upset with him because he had not finished copying his spelling words. We also observed that Mitch's earlier difficulties with printing were gone. Although he wrote slowly, he was able to stay on the line, and his letters were readable. We also observed that Mitch was probably the quietest child in the room. He seldom talked to any other child, although he watched other children closely, and often imitated what he saw them doing. Observation in the Chapter I classroom confirmed that Mitch did experience more success with reading in that environment. The teacher worked with groups of four or five children at a time, and she gave much more individual instruction. She used trade books organized around themes chosen by the children themselves. Mitch's father was a construction worker, and he had chosen to read books about "building things." Because he was interested, and because he had a good deal of background knowledge to bring to the reading enterprise, he was experiencing some success. The Chapter I teacher confirmed, however, that while he might guess about what a word ought to be in the context, he had no ability to sound out words he didn't recognize.

The focused testing of Mitch was completed during March of his first grade year. Because of Mitch's problems with syntax and morphology as a preschooler, we decided to test his knowledge of syntax and morphology. The CELF-R was administered. This testing yielded the following standard scores (the mean standard score is 10; a score of 7 is 1 standard deviation below the mean):

Receptive Language Score	74
Expressive Language Score	67
Total Language Score	69
Oral Directions	4
Word Classes	6
Semantic Relationships	8
Formulated Sentences	3
Recalling Sentences	7
Sentence Assembly	5
Listening to Paragraphs	4
Word Associations	7
Linguistic Concepts	6

The Receptive, Expressive, and Total Language Scores are more than one standard deviation below the mean. In fact the Expressive Score and Total Score are more than two standard deviations below the mean. The difference between the Receptive and Expressive Scores is not significant. The only subtest scores that fell within one standard deviation of the mean were Semantic Relationships, Recalling Sentences, and Word Associations. These results confirmed what we had observed about Mitch's ability to follow directions. On the Oral Directions subtest, Mitch did well until the instructions began to involve complex relational terms, such as "Point to the small circle on the right of the black triangle." With instructions such as these, Mitch appeared to respond at random, and made it clear that he did not want to continue the task.

The informal testing of metalinguistic abilities showed major problems in this area. Mitch was unable to respond with consistent accuracy to questions about "how many sounds are in this word". Even after several practice items, he acted as though he was not sure what he was being asked to do. In the phoneme elision task, when he had to tell what would be left when, for example, we took the "s" sound away from "sit," he responded correctly to 50% of the questions about taking off the initial sound, but could not respond to questions involving taking off the final sound. He responded with 80% accuracy to a task involving telling whether words rhymed. He seemed to be confused if the final sounds of the words were different, saying, for example, that "heat" and "heap" rhymed. The four children from his classroom, who were described by the teacher as "right in the middle of the class," had no difficulty at all with any of the phonological awareness tasks. Given that they had all had a year of phonics instruction in kindergarten and half a year in first grade, they probably were more advanced in this area than children their age without formal instruction, but since these were the children Mitch was being compared with in school, the discrepancy in the test results was of great concern.

We consulted with Mitch's teacher to decide what event the members of his class might have in common, so we could gather several recountings of the event to compare. She suggested that we ask the children to tell about a recent trip to the supermarket to buy ingredients for a meal. An analysis of the narrative sample indicated that Mitch's attempt to tell about this scripted event lacked cohesion and organization. He tended to give much more information than was necessary about some points, such as the automated checkout, and no information at all about other points, such as the fact that they had made up a list in advance and were trying to find the items on the list. These difficulties with presupposition and organization resulted in a narrative that seemed to have no point. The other four children from his classroom who participated in this task gave recountings of varied lengths, but of generally coherent organization. Rather than going into detail about specific aspects of the event, they all gave the general framework of "We made up a grocery list for an imaginary lunch with spaghetti and salad and bread and we went to the store to find the things on our list. We went all over the store to find all the things. We had to wait in line at the checkout and the teacher paid for the food." Since this event recounting had been developed in the classroom after the event, it was not surprising that the four "average" children gave roughly the same account. However, this made Mitch's account seem all the more inadequate.

On a story retelling task, Mitch demonstrated very little story grammar. His attempt tended to describe the pictures rather than tell the story. The story we gave Mitch to retell contained five episodes, and he was unable to recount any complete episodes. Based on previous testing of many first grade children in Mitch's school on this task, we know that the average first grader can complete at least 50% of the episodes in this story, and many first graders can retell all of the episodes. Mitch's failure to retell the story with any of the narrative structure intact was clearly inadequate.

It was difficult to obtain a conversational language sample of any length from Mitch, because of his reticence. He tended to reply to questions with the briefest possible responses, and did not initiate topics himself. However, Mitch had told his teacher that his cat had had kittens, and he had seemed very animated about this. Since Mitch's mother picked him up every day from school, we asked her to bring in the mother cat and kittens in a box, so Mitch could tell his teacher about them. We tape recorded Mitch's conversation with his teacher as they admired the kittens, and Mitch talked about what they had been named and what kinds of things they did. In analyzing this conversation, we discovered that Mitch consistently talked as though the teacher knew everything he knew, indicating inappropriate presuppositions. He was also prone to drift away from the topic, as though he were "free associating."

In looking at all the data from our observation and testing, we concluded that Mitch continued to demonstrate a language disorder. The results of the classroom observation and the concerns expressed by the teacher indicated the strong possibility that Mitch's academic progress was being affected by his language difficulty. In other words, Mitch's first grade classroom demanded a level of phonological awareness sufficient to allow him to handle phonics instruction. Mitch's phonological awareness was well below that of other children in the classroom, and insufficient to allow him to deal with phonics instruction. Mitch's reading comprehension will be affected by his knowledge of narrative structure and his ability to use event frameworks to aid recall and organization. His ability to use a story grammar framework in a story retelling task was substantially below that of other children in first grade. In addition, scripted event recountings are among the most common, and usually the easiest expressive language tasks for school-aged children. Mitch's expressive language use on this task was inadequate, particularly when compared with that of other children in the classroom. His conversational meaning was often lost due to his problems with presupposition and topic maintenance. The intervention goals we established based on this case will be discussed in Chapter 2.

Case 2. Jackie: The Child Identified as Language Impaired After Starting School

Jackie was a beautiful little girl, with long red ringlets. When we first saw her, she was dressed in a yellow dress, and the lace on her socks matched the ribbon in her hair. Her teacher reported that she lived with her mother and grandmother, and that "they treat her like a little doll." It was clear that she was a loved, confident child. She was quite willing to talk with the speech-language pathologist, and walked into the room and sat down at the table in a composed fashion. Jackie had been referred by the learning disabilities teacher for assessment because she had transferred into the school with a diagnosis of "learning disabled" which had been made while she was in second grade. Jackie was receiving 1 ½ hours of learning resource classroom instruction daily. She was reading at a first grade level, in spite of two years of Whole Language classroom instruction. Her second grade teacher had reported that Jackie had great difficulty following directions in the classroom. She said, "she isn't a bad child in any way. She just seems to be lost most of the time." In addition, the teacher wondered whether Jackie might have "some kind of problem with understanding" since she frequently failed to answer questions in class, and seemed "to get lost in the middle of things she is trying to tell you." In addition, Jackie was reported to have problems with concepts of measurement, time, and money, although her math computation skills were normal. Her math skills were being monitored in the learning resources classroom.

After only a few weeks of working with Jackie, the learning resources teacher suggested that the speech-language pathologist evaluate her. The teacher had noticed several similarities between Jackie and other children who were language impaired, including some apparent difficulties with specific vocabulary, as seen in the conversation below:

Clinician: Can you tell me what you do in swimming class?
Jackie: Well, first you have to put on your swimming suit and you walk under that thing with the water, you know, where you get wet. Then you go through this other place where you have to walk through this water that smells kind of funny. That's so you won't get germs on your feet. Then the teacher tells us to get in the water, and we have to hold onto our things and kick our feet a lot. And when you have to put your face in the water, you can get it in your eyes. Some people have these things on their eyes, you know, these [PUTS HER FINGERS AROUND HER EYES TO INDICATE GLASSES].
Clinician: Goggles, you mean?
Jackie: Yeah, those. And if you want to, you can put stuff in your ears so water won't get in, and then you won't get hurting in your ears. And then

we have to hold those things, you know, those flat things [OUTLINES A SHAPE WITH HER HANDS].
Clinician: Do they call those float boards?
Jackie: Yeah, those boards, and we kick some more.

Jackie was able to talk in a reasonably organized way about her swimming lessons. She also talked willingly about what she liked most about school (art), and her sentence structure and vocabulary in the course of conversation seemed quite appropriate. However, as the resource teacher noted, she frequently struggled to come up with specific vocabulary words, and resorted to gestures or general words such as "thing." In addition, the resource teacher reported that Jackie seemed to have particular problems with class directions. She would complete part of an assignment, and not even attempt the rest. Sometimes she acted as though she had only heard the first part or the last part of what she was expected to do, and had "blanked out" the middle.

Jackie's mother reported no problems with her language development as a preschooler. She also saw no problems with Jackie's language as a second grader, and confessed that she thought Jackie's problems with reading were largely the teacher's fault. In fact, in casual conversation, anyone might have failed to find any problems with Jackie's language. Her very observant teacher had zeroed in on two of the biggest problems: she had great difficulty with auditory memory, and in addition her spontaneous language use suggested a probable word-finding difficulty, which might have contributed to her slowness to answer questions in class.

> Word finding disorders are characterized by the inability to retrieve specific words, even when these words are known. It is not a vocabulary problem. The child has the vocabulary, and can use it in some contexts, or retrieve it with particular cues.

Although every individual child will come with his or her own set of strengths and weaknesses, Jackie's set of problems is not atypical of those seen in children who are referred by observant or perplexed classroom teachers. She was fine in social settings, and her coping skills served her well in those situations. However, when confronted with the need to retrieve specific vocabulary, or to recall specific sequences of spoken instructions, she fell apart. In addition, in a classroom which focused on reading as a skill involving predicting meaning rather than decoding words, she was having difficulty learning to read. Jackie's problems seemed to be involved not so much with learning language as with using language to learn. This set of problems certainly suggests a need for some focused assessment.

Clinical Brainstorming: Jackie

We had less information about Jackie's development of language than we had about Mitch's. Jackie had transferred into the school at the beginning of third grade, having been classified Learning Disabled as a second grader. (As we did in Mitch's case, we have included relevant documents from Jackie's cumulative file in Appendix 1.) This classification was based on the severe discrepancy between her IQ, which was average, and her achievement, which was two years below grade level in reading. The learning disabilities teacher, who was very aware of language impairment, suggested that Jackie should be tested. Her description suggested that Jackie might have a word-finding problem and possibly some auditory memory problems as well.

Ann: I always wonder, when people talk about a child having a memory problem, whether we're dealing with a storage problem or a retrieval problem. I think most people assume that a memory problem is automatically a storage problem—that information just doesn't stick. When you think about it though, much of the behavior we see, such as not being able to remember someone's name, could as easily be ascribed to retrieval problems.

Rita: You're right. How do we decide which is which?

Ann: I'm not sure we are always able to. But in this case, we need to make every effort to determine whether Jackie really knows some of the vocabulary she isn't using. In other words, does she have a problem learning new vocabulary, in the sense that it takes lots of exposure before the word and the meaning stick in her brain together, or is it that she just can't seem to pull up the label when she needs to?

Rita: I agree with you. I suspect that Jackie has had problems with people thinking she didn't know material that she, in fact, knew quite well but just couldn't talk about. What I also worry about is her difficulty following directions. I wonder whether she's having some general problem holding information in working memory long enough to act on it. I guess we'd better do some general testing there. The *Detroit Test of Learning Abilities*-3 (Detroit-3; Hammill, 1991) has some good subtests for looking at verbal memory.

Debbie: We also need to find out whether her memory for visual sequences is the same, or whether visual input helps her. The Detroit-3 will also have visual memory subtests.

Rita: If we are dealing with some memory difficulties, we need to find out what kinds of frameworks Jackie might have to help structure material for memory. For example, is it easier for her to recall information when it's presented in a story framework? Sometimes, the knowledge of narrative structure helps the child predict, and predictability will help remembering. Let's do a story retelling task with her. [Story retelling tasks are described in Chapter 5.]

Debbie: Even if she's having difficulty decoding words when she reads, it may be that reading will be a better way for her to get information. Listening may be too hard for her. I'd also like to investigate her ability to work on an "idea map." You know, when you read a story about a little girl who planted a garden, and after the story, you and the child construct a map of everything the child knows about "gardens." Some children can use this as a help in comprehending a story, because it helps them bring their real-world knowledge to bear. Other children seem to have real problems doing this. They can tell you only a few things about the key concept, and then they seem to run out of steam. If Jackie can do this kind of thing, it might be a strategy to help her with reading. [The use of idea maps and other graphic organizers is discussed in Chapter 8.]

Rita: I'd like to observe her in peer groups in less structured situations. Her social skills look good, but I'd like to see her with her friends. I want to know how well she holds her own in a conversation or a discussion when several children are competing for time, and it's not just one-on-one.

Ann: Let's summarize. I want a hearing screening, even though nobody has ever suggested problems. Let's just be certain. We want to do some observation, both in the classroom and in the peer group. Then we need to take a look at auditory and visual memory. We'll give the Detroit-3. Then, let's give the CELF-R, to compare her performance on the subtests requiring auditory memory with those not requiring this ability. Then, to take a look at the word finding, we can give the *Test of Word Finding* (German, 1986). There's a comprehension section that will give us some insight into her receptive vocabulary, and there's a confrontation naming task. I'd like to find out whether giving her an "either/or" choice will trigger a response when she has a word finding problem. Then we want to find out about her narrative abilities. Can she tell a story to a wordless picture book? How does she do with a story retelling task? And when we do a shared book reading, can she predict logical outcomes or make inferences using context clues? What kind of idea map can she generate after hearing a story? Story frameworks and inferencing abilities will relate to her reading comprehension abilities.

Results of the assessment

Our observation of Jackie in the classroom and on the playground confirmed our first impression of her. She was socially adept and confident. She seemed to have two or three "best friends" with whom she played most of the time. She was a leader in this small group, usually being the one who decided what they would do. Although her word finding difficulties were apparent to an adult listener, her animated use of gesture and her circumlocutions seemed to cause no difficulty for her in social interactions. In the larger classroom group, she was somewhat more reticent, but not unduly so. Her word finding difficulties sometimes caused her to seem unassertive when the teacher asked for volunteers to answer questions. She seldom raised her hand unless the answer was a "yes/no" or other either/or choice which did not demand that she retrieve specific vocabulary. If the teacher did call on her for a specific answer, she simply replied "I don't know," or, occasionally, "I can't think of it."

On the story retelling task, she showed no awareness of narrative structure. Her retelling consisted entirely of descriptions of the pictures. She also failed to repeat any dialogue from the story, in contrast to the usual performance of other children her age. Her response to the wordless picture book also consisted of picture descriptions, with no story structure. We used the Mercer Meyer book called *A Boy, a Dog, and a Frog*, and Jackie's "story" was as follows:

> He's a frog, and he's running. See, he got [elaborate gestures]. And then he said "hi, frog." And then he jumped in the water. Then he jumps and went like this [elaborate gestures of swimming]. Then he caught the dog, and the frog jumped in the water. Then he said "I'll get you, frog." Then they went [gestures trying to catch the frog] and he tried to catch the frog. And then he followed their footprints like this [acts out frog hopping along]. Then he followed and followed, and he's in the bathtub. Then he jumps [acts out frog jumping].

For comparison purposes, Jackie's best friend from her classroom, Lisa, was asked to tell a story to the same wordless picture book. Part of her story (which was quite long), is given below:

> The boy's going fishing, and he's looking for some water nearby. Instead, he sees a frog. He wants to get that frog and take it home. He tries to get the frog, but he lands headfirst in the water and the frog gets mad. And when he came out of the water, he was looking straight at the frog. The frog jumped onto a log. The boy said to the dog, "You go to that side of the log and I'll go to the other." They tried to sneak up on the frog. The dog got there first. He tried to grab the frog, and the frog hopped off and caught the dog. The boy got mad, and marched away, dragging his nets behind. The frog was sad. [etc., etc.]

When we read a story with Jackie (*Tacky the Penguin* by Helen Lester), stopping to ask inferencing questions such as "Why are they throwing rocks at those guys?" or logical reasoning questions, such as "How do they know there's a storm coming?" Jackie could answer the reasoning questions if the information needed was present in a picture (they knew a storm was coming because there was a big black cloud with lightning coming out of it), but she could not explain that the boys were throwing rocks at the three men because they were trying to frighten them away. The picture showed the rock throwing, and the text simply said "They tried all kinds of ways to frighten the men away." When we tried to generate an idea map with Jackie, around the story episode in which the penguins try to frighten away the hunters, Jackie was able to come up with only two ideas about what kinds of things a person would do to frighten away an enemy ("get a gun and point it at him" and "call the police"). She seemed to have great difficulty putting herself in the place of the book's characters who were threatened and trying to frighten away the source of the threat.

On the *Test of Word Finding*, Jackie's comprehension score was 98%, indicating that she did understand the vocabulary used on this test. The results of the assessment indicated that Jackie was a "slow and inaccurate namer." Her responses were frequently accompanied by extra verbalizations such as "um" and gestures, sometimes very elaborate gestures. These results indicate that Jackie could be expected to take an appreciably longer time to respond to teacher requests than her peers and that her responses were less likely to be correct. In fact this corresponds to the observations of the classroom teacher and the speech-language pathologist. Further analysis of Jackie's responses indicated that most of her incorrect responses were Superordinate (naming the semantic class in place of the target word), Functional Attributes (the word given represents a function of the target word), or Circumlocutions (multi-word substitutions for the target word).

The memory testing presented us with a more complicated picture. it was clear to us that Jackie had difficulty holding linguistic input in her working memory. We administered the entire CELF-R to Jackie, so we would have some basis for comparing her performance on subtests requiring auditory memory and subtests not requiring so much memory use. Her scores were:

Oral Directions	3
Word Classes	10
Semantic Relationships	10
Formulated Sentences	10
Recalling Sentences	4
Sentence Assembly	13
Listening to Paragraphs	3
Word Associations	6
Linguistic Concepts	10

On this test, Jackie had difficulty remembering factual information from the paragraphs we read to her. She could usually recall information from the beginning of the paragraph, but nothing more. She could not imitate any sentence more than 5 words long. Other subtests on the CELF-R show Jackie performing at or slightly above the mean, but subtests requiring auditory memory were significantly below the mean. The results of the Detroit-3 showed that her auditory memory for sentences and paragraphs was well below average, while her visual memory was average to slightly above average for her age.

We concluded that in addition to her learning disability, Jackie had a communication impairment that was contributing to her academic difficulties. Her auditory memory for linguistic material was one obvious part of the problem, as was her difficulty with word finding. We knew that narrative frameworks would be important to help Jackie structure material she heard or read, and we were alarmed to see that she gave no evidence of having a story grammar framework in her retelling or in her own story generated to pictures. She had difficulty answering inferencing questions about the story, and was unable to bring her own real-world knowledge to bear in talking about a story episode. As the school curriculum places greater demands on Jackie's ability to use language to learn, these problems with using narrative framework will become critical elements in Jackie's academic performance. The intervention goals we established on the basis of this evaluation will be discussed in Chapter 2.

SUMMARY

In this chapter, we have laid the groundwork for a clinical approach to language impairment in school-aged children. We have rejected a discrepancy definition of language impairment, first because we believe such definitions cause unhealthy reliance on test scores which provide a narrow picture of the child's language abilities, and second, because such definitions ignore the child's ability to function in the communication context of the classroom and the peer group. Of equal importance in our decision to set aside such a definition is the increasing recognition that discrepancy based definitions of language impairment do not seem to match very well with clinical judgments in the field, and we are unwilling to set aside the informed judgment of experienced clinicians. This mismatch may be due in part to the fact that available standardized tests focus on phonology, morphology, syntax, and vocabulary in isolation from any communicative context. They do not assess the higher level language processes the child needs to function in the classroom and to become literate. Informed clinicians know this, and have developed other methods of assessing children which provide them with the kinds of information they need about the child's language use.

Our own clinical approach to language impairment starts from perspective of the child's functioning in the environment. A child who is experiencing academic problems or serious difficulty in a peer group **because of difficulties with language** is, in our view, language impaired and in need of services. We have outlined a practical approach to deciding whether children's academic or social problems have their roots in language functioning. The key words in our approach are: **focus, observe, think,** and only after this, **test.** Having made the determination that a particular child is language impaired, the speech-language pathologist in the school is faced with the necessity to plan intervention. The intervention context will be the focus of Chapter 2, as we continue to follow the cases of Mitch and Jackie.

C H A P T E R 2

The Real World of Collaborative, Classroom Based Language Intervention

In this chapter, we will introduce you to the principles and practices of collaborative, curriculum based intervention for children with language impairments. We will begin by defining two key terms, and then move to a description of how Marilyn, the school speech-language pathologist introduced in Chapter 1, established her program. You will follow her through the process of setting up a collaborative, curriculum based model, as she moved away from a traditional approach to intervention. Then we will provide a description of a typical day for Marilyn, and establish the intervention principles which govern such a program. Finally, we will return to the cases of Mitch and Jackie presented in Chapter 1, develop Individual Education Plans for each student, and provide some samples of typical intervention lessons.

DEFINITIONS OF KEY TERMS

Two terms will appear repeatedly throughout this chapter and the intervention chapters which follow it. These are **collaboration** and **classroom based intervention**. For more than 50 years, speech language intervention in the schools has been based on a "pull out" model. We take the child out of the classroom and walk down a long hallway to a very small room to conduct "speech therapy" or "speech class." For some children this was and is an appropriate model. However, what was done in the "therapy room" often had very little if any relevance to what the child was doing in the classroom. When we took the child back to his classroom, his classmates were either deeply involved in a learning activity or had moved on to something else. In either case our child had no idea what was going on. However, his teacher and his classmates expected him to know and to fit right into the classroom milieu. Every school speech-language pathologist can tell a sad story like this one from a clinician of our acquaintance: "I will never forget the child who started to cry during my therapy session for no apparent reason. With gentle questioning, I found out that he was missing math class and that his teacher was going to keep him out of recess so that he could make up the math lesson he was missing." Surely there is a better way to work with children and to collaborate with teachers.

Many school speech-language pathologists have also tried to involve classroom teachers in the therapy procedure for the child. We would try to catch teachers in the lounge, or during planning time, or before or after school and tell them what we were working on and what they could do to help with "carry over." Teachers usually listened very patiently and some even tried hard to provide the feedback that we requested. Usually, however, they could not see that what went on in "speech" had anything to do with what went on in their classrooms. We were, in effect, adding to their burdens when we asked them to help us.

Now we realize that the child with a language/learning difficulty is already having trouble seeing the relationship among the lessons and activities in the classroom, and taking him out of that classroom three or four times a day for resource work doesn't help. He may have difficulty dealing with the pragmatics of the classroom or he may have difficulty following directions, but whatever his problem is, removing him from the classroom situation and working on things that do not (to him) have any readily apparent relationship to classroom activities makes his life even more disjointed and disconnected. How much better and more meaningful for the child if we tailor our treatment to what is happening in the classroom. This, **classroom based intervention**, does not necessarily mean that the speech-language pathologist is in the classroom teaching with the teacher, although there are times when this might be an appropriate activity. It means that wherever the intervention service is provided, even in the little therapy room, the treatment is built around or supplements the lessons being taught in the classroom. This model requires that the speech-language pathologist should know something about all the curricula in her school. It also requires that the clinician think in terms of learning strategies rather than content areas.

For example, what strategies does the child need in order to gain information from his textbook, whether the subject matter is social studies,

Each school district has grade level curriculum guides, which have been developed by teachers to meet state and national education standards in all areas of academics. Broad-based goals and objectives are set within each area to provide a framework for teachers to build their curriculums. Check with the school principal or librarian for the location of the curriculum guides for your district. In addition, contact your state department of education for statewide proficiency guides.

math, or science? It requires that the clinician learn to see how language impairment is reflected in the child's academic success or failure. Basically, then, the classroom based intervention model (also referred to as curriculum based) means that we look at the child's communication strengths and weaknesses and identify how those strengths and weaknesses affect success in the classroom. Then we tailor our intervention plan to provide the child the opportunity to develop his skills so that he is better able to learn in the classroom. If we are successful, the child will be successful as well, and academic success will be within reach.

In order to operate a classroom based intervention program it is essential to develop **collaboration** among all the school personnel involved in the child's programming. Collaboration implies a partnership. The speech-language pathologist has valuable information to offer to the classroom teacher. We have training and experience in analyzing a child's behavior in communication contexts and in helping the child develop strategies to improve communication skills. The classroom teacher has expertise in classroom management and knowledge about the curriculum that most speech-language pathologists lack. By combining the two bodies of information it is possible to implement a powerful intervention program. But it is essential that the speech-language pathologist view herself as a part of a team; as a collaborator, not as a consultant. A consultant looks over the situation and then tells everyone what should be done. A collaborator talks over the situation, getting everyone's perspective, including her own, out on the table. The entire group then works to derive and implement an appropriate solution. This model is new to many speech-language pathologists and classroom teachers alike. We must understand that we as speech-language pathologists are not the only ones who can work on language. Language is an integral part of every classroom. We need to help the classroom teacher recognize the communication/language environment and how to manage it to meet the needs of the special child. In doing this, both we and the teacher may recognize strategies that will benefit all the children in the classroom, not just those who are language impaired.

ESTABLISHING A NEW KIND OF PROGRAM

Statement of Principle: As speech-language pathologists we must work to develop intervention programs which meet the needs of today's language impaired students. We cannot and should not develop or implement these programs alone. Through collaboration with school personnel and parents we will learn about the whole child and how his or her language deficits impact the quality of the school experience. Entering the classroom for most students will have many positive outcomes. We must continue to evaluate current practices, reflect on their strengths and weaknesses, and challenge ourselves to become members of a team which addresses the needs of students using progressive strategies.

Moving Toward Change: Year 1

(The story you are about to read is true. Only the names have been changed, to protect the privacy of the individuals involved.) Marilyn was a speech-language pathologist for a rural school system in the Midwest. The system enrolled a high proportion of children from poverty. Six years ago, when she began work in this school system, she inherited a traditional schedule and caseload from the previous clinician. She was assigned to provide services to two elementary schools. In common with most school SLPs at that time, she decided to divide her time equally between the schools, spending two and one half days at each. Her therapy exemplified the traditional pull-out process in wide practice at the time. The children loved to come to "Speech," but Marilyn soon realized that there was little relationship between what children did in her room and what they did in the classroom.

She soon became frustrated with this situation. As she learned more about grade-level expectations, classroom environments, literacy development, and the school schedule, it became clear to her that there had to be a better way. Many of the children in the school who were "normal" were having trouble meeting the demands of the classroom, and those children in her caseload with language problems frequently failed altogether. Whatever she was doing in language therapy, she reasoned, wasn't helping the children in the classroom. Whether this was due to a failure to achieve carryover, or whether her language goals were irrelevant to the child's school work was not clear. She was particularly frustrated that the teaching staff knew very little about what she was doing, and seemed to care even less. The parents of children in her caseload also had little understanding of what the goals were for their children, and did not associate the "speech" goals with anything that was going on in the classroom. Sometimes parents even expressed concern that a child would be missing something "important" in the classroom when he went for "speech."

One day, in conversation with a building principal, the entire situation was crystallized for her. The principal said to her, "You are working in a school, not in a speech clinic. You need to look at the bigger picture." Of course, she was correct. The speech-language services were not an integral part of any student's educational plan, the bigger picture. They were written into the IEP, but the goals and the intervention plan were isolated from the rest of the child's educational program. The child was not benefitting in any real-life sense.

Through her continuing education efforts, Marilyn learned about the concepts of a collaborative model and classroom-based intervention. The philosophy behind the collaborative model is that a team of professionals with different skills and perspectives is more likely to provide an evaluation of a student's strengths and weaknesses from the perspective of the whole child rather than from a series of individual professional viewpoints. The collaborative model provides for a team to evaluate the student, develop an educational plan, implement the plan, evaluate progress, and modify the plan as needed throughout the school year. "Great idea," thought Marilyn. "But before I can get anything like this started, I have to start talking to the other people who are working with the children in my caseload." With this thought, Marilyn began to make a determined effort to talk with the other special education professionals in her schools. She talked at lunch, at recess, and after school. She asked to see records and reports. She offered to share information. Not everyone was open and ready for this initially, but Marilyn soon found that there were people like her, feeling frustrated by the fragmentation of the children's programs and by their own professional isolation.

Classroom-based intervention was also appealing to Marilyn. The philosophy behind classroom-based intervention is that language learning is intrinsic to literacy development. The approach uses the student's grade level curriculum as a context for intervention. The curriculum is modified as needed by the team and the student is taught specific strategies which enable access to critical content. "How much more relevant could I get," Marilyn said to herself. "If the materials I use in therapy are taken directly from the child's classroom, and if the goals are directly related to what the child needs to be able to do to succeed in the classroom, maybe I'll begin to see carryover."

Moving Toward Change: Year 2

Statement of Principle: Oral and written language are the primary means by which children demonstrate what they have learned within the school environment.

During her second year in the district, Marilyn's schedule did not look remarkably different from the way it had looked the first year. However, what was happening in her treatment sessions was noticeably different. Marilyn attended workshops and read journal articles about the connection between communicative competency and school success. She watched and talked with the few teachers in her schools doing language based instruction. It became clear to Marilyn that oral and written language were the crux of all learning. Then one day a first grade student enrolled in language therapy brought a book with him to share during his session. Marilyn saw an opportunity to use the book as a basis for the language lesson she had planned. When he left 30 minutes later, she realized that this had been the most meaningful language intervention she had provided in some time. Suddenly there was a shared, natural context to a lesson. Marilyn and the child talked about the sequence of events in the book, concentrating on vocabulary to communicate about time, such as "before," "after," and "while." When the child returned to the classroom, it was natural and appropriate for the teacher to ask questions which provided the child with opportunities to review, recall, or retell the story they had worked on in "speech class." Marilyn reflected, "As always, I continue to learn from my students."

Marilyn was still faced with a serious concern. The fourth, fifth, and sixth grade children who were seen by both the SLP and the resource teacher were failing in all content areas. This led her to study the textbooks used by these children in science and social studies. It became evident that some of the vocabulary and text constructions were extremely difficult for the language impaired children. Marilyn began to help the teachers identify the areas where language impaired children would have particular problems. It wasn't long before the classroom teachers learned to rely on the SLP to help them identify the parts of the text they needed to give extra help with. Marilyn then began to focus her intervention on text structures that were problematic for the children across all content areas. For example, most of the children in her caseload were completely unable to find the main idea of a paragraph or a chapter. When attempting to summarize what they had read, they were as likely to focus on irrelevant detail as on important information. Marilyn's focus was always on strategies for gleaning information from the text, and for taking tests, and for completing class projects, not on the specifics of any content area.

The teachers reported that the children were improving in their participation in class. As the SLP shared with the classroom teachers the kinds of difficulties language impaired children were having with the textbook, the teachers came to realize that perhaps other children were having similar difficulties. For example, in reviewing the text and helping one language impaired child prepare for his test, Marilyn asked the child to list the advantages and disadvantages of a particular process. It became immediately clear to her that the child did not know the words "advantage" and "disadvantage," and that he did not understand how to compare and contrast. When Marilyn discussed this with the teacher, they decided together that Marilyn should provide a mini-lesson for the entire class about these words, and about the idea of comparing and contrasting. This first mini-lesson in a classroom was a real breakthrough for Marilyn, for the teacher, and for the children in the class. Marilyn began to see the possibilities of the model she was struggling with.

While her second year was an improvement over the first year, it still fell short of her vision for the program. While she was planning for ways to change even more, PL 99-457 was implemented in her state, and preschool classrooms became Marilyn's responsibility. Marilyn immediately saw that the preschool classrooms gave her an opportunity to enter into classroom activity up-front, rather than through the back door. She could work on facilitating children's communication in their everyday classroom environments, because she was mandated to do so!

Moving Toward Change: Year 3

Statement of Principle: Every school district has a process for evaluating and assisting children who are experiencing academic difficulties. Some of those children may be language impaired. It is the responsibility of the school speech-language pathologist to educate school personnel about the impact a language impairment can have on academic and social success. A speech-language pathologist should always be considered as part of the multidisciplinary team assembled to gather information about a student experiencing academic and/or social failure and develop an individual education plan to meet the special needs of the student.

Marilyn's schedule for the third year began to reflect some of the changes in philosophy about language evaluation, intervention, and caseload selection she had made in the previous year. She noted that the governing provision for Special Education services in her state held that a child must demonstrate impairments that affected either social or academic performance in order to qualify for services. In the previous two years, Marilyn had enrolled on her caseload first and second grade children who were exhibiting one or two sound errors, but whose speech was intelligible. Fourth, fifth, or sixth grade students were also enrolled if they had lingering single phoneme articulation errors due to lack of carryover outside the therapy room. Usually, these articulation difficulties were brought to the attention of the parents, teachers, and the student by Marilyn herself. The articulation "problem" was usually not adversely affecting the student's educational performance in any way. Marilyn decided to use the state law as an impetus for taking a closer look at her caseload.

She was able to identify a few children in the upper elementary grades who experienced teasing from the peer group because of an /r/ distortion, or whose parents wanted the child's /s/ corrected. At the case conferences for these children, she made it clear that she would teach the student to produce to phoneme at the word and sentence level with 85% accuracy in the therapy room. Carryover would be the responsibility of the student and the family. This approach resulted in several children being dismissed from the caseload, giving Marilyn more hours per week to reallocate than she had previously had.

In her previous schedules, Marilyn had only limited time for collaborative assessment. Time was needed to observe the child in the classroom during key periods during the day. Time was needed to interview the teacher(s), review cumulative records, read reports from the school psychologist, occupational therapist, or school nurse. Time was needed to observe the child at recess, at lunch, or in gym class. Only after gathering all the available information would Marilyn be ready to determine what questions needed to be answered about the child's communication abilities and what standardized or clinician constructed assessment procedures would be most appropriate to answer those questions. Somehow, Marilyn had to find the time to do this right.

Since preschool services were now being offered in the school buildings, and these children were added to Marilyn's caseload, she needed to do some serious thinking about how to find time for that as well. Marilyn found that the teacher in the preschool classroom was a licensed early intervention special educator. Her classroom was language based and provided a wonderful natural environment for communication development. She found that spending an hour and 30 minutes in the morning class, and an hour in the afternoon class once a week, gave the teacher the support she needed to help them both meet the goals and objectives that they had developed collaboratively. The preschool classroom assistant carried out articulation lesson plans, assembled communication boards, and kept track of student progress in a log. As long as the SLP provided the goals and objectives, and shared teaching strategies, the teacher and assistant were highly capable of assisting in the implementation of a speech and language program in the classroom. Marilyn's weekly schedule in year 3 looked like this:

Monday and Wednesday: School A all day
Tuesday and Friday: School B all day
Thursday: 7:45–9:15 School C (Preschool)
9:15–9:45 Travel
10:00–12:00 Diagnostics or Conferences (where needed)
12:00–12:30 Lunch
12:30–1:45 Diagnostics or Conferences (continued)
1:45–2:15 Travel
2:15–3:15 School C (Preschool)

This schedule addressed many of Marilyn's concerns. She was by now an integral part of the collaborative assessment team. Very rarely was a child seen for assessment by the school psychologist that Marilyn did not know it. She was a member of the pre-assessment committee, which met with the school psychologist when a child was referred by a teacher. However, some problems remained. There was no planning time, no record or report writing time, and certainly no set time for collaboration with teachers. Most of these activities occurred after school or over the telephone on weekends. This situation needed to be changed! Back to the drawing board with the schedule.

Marilyn designed a final schedule to keep herself in one school for a longer period of time during the week. It allowed time for diagnostic testing, therapy services, hearing screening, report writing, record keeping, and team meetings and planning time with teachers. Marilyn set up a schedule which alternated by weeks rather than by days. This schedule was as follows, with her week at a particular school beginning on a Thursday.

Week 1

Thursday:	Elementary School A and School C (preschool)
Friday:	Elementary School A
Monday:	Elementary School A
Tuesday:	Elementary School A
Wednesday:	Elementary School A

Week 2

Thursday:	Elementary School B and School C (preschool)
Friday:	Elementary School B and School C (preschool)
Monday:	Elementary School B
Tuesday:	Elementary School B
Wednesday:	Elementary School B

As you can see, this new schedule met the needs of her changing program by minimizing travel time between schools and maximizing her ability to focus on the needs of the students and teachers in a particular location. It is important to understand how her daily schedule throughout the week differed as well. Thursday and Friday were divided between the preschool classroom, evaluations, team meetings, conferences, and collaborative planning with teachers. Monday, Tuesday, and Wednesday were spent providing therapy services. Having three consecutive days for therapy in a location proved very effective for students since most thematic classroom activities spanned several days. What follows is a description of some typical school days taken from Marilyn's diary. It should give you a better idea of just how a typical week unfolds.

A DAY IN THE LIFE

Monday – Wednesday

7:45 — Meet with student with oral motor problems in the cafeteria and practice chewing exercises while he eats breakfast. Tomorrow will see him in the speech-language room to focus on lip closure using words associated with current classroom themes.

8:00 — Meet with a language impaired fourth grader (and two classmates) in the library to work on "place value" concepts as well as coach him in a search for five facts about pioneers to record in his state history journal.

8:30 — Meet with three language impaired students in their first grade classroom to coach them through completion of a "cut and paste" project associated with a story that was read earlier that morning by the classroom teacher. (We will discuss the "oral directions" given by the teacher and the "problem" in the story read earlier.)

9:00 — Meet with two language impaired students in another first grade classroom. The class has been divided into groups for a "nature walk." My group (2 language impaired, 3 normal) predicts what we will see outdoors. We discuss our ideas verbally and then make a list together. We talk about "words" and "sounds." the kids take a clipboard outside and write what they see. The language impaired kids take a tape recorder and tell what they see. Later in the week we write their ideas on paper as we recount the event.

9:30 — Go into the kindergarten classroom where they are discussing "Emergencies." The class is divided into 3 groups to practice a "calling 911" script. My group (and the classroom assistant's group) has all language normal children and is larger than the classroom teacher's group which contains one hearing impaired child, one child with emotional problems, one child with articulation problems, and two "normal" children. (We take turns working with the disabled students so that we can all talk intelligently about their needs and progress.)

10:00 — Meet with a language impaired fifth grade student with good decoding skills but poor reading comprehension skills, during the "silent reading" portion of her language arts period. The class is focusing on understanding "character development." We look for selected words, phrases, and sentences which may give clues about the characters. We discuss how she might describe herself if she were a character in a story.

10:30 — Meet with four language impaired students with significant auditory processing difficulties and decoding problems in reading. We go to the library and find several picture books about pioneers. The students decide to write their own book called *Wild, Wild Pioneers*. We talk about a plan for developing the book and write it down. I write a quick note to the resource teacher suggesting she use this activity as the context for her lessons later in the week.

11:00 — Go to a second grade classroom with the special education resource teacher. There are five language impaired/learning disabled students in this class. We present a lesson on story grammar to the whole class. The children listen to a simple story read aloud and then we discuss the "problem" in the story, what caused the "problem" and how the characters tried to solve the "problem.

11:30 — Lunch with teachers to discuss writing a grant proposal.

12:00 — Call about Student Assistance team meeting schedule at other building.

12:15 — Go into sixth grade social studies class. Observe whether a language impaired/LD student is implementing the text strategies she knows to answer questions related to the chapter being studied.

12:45 — Go into kindergarten classroom during "area time" and observe a student whose language and play skills the classroom teacher is concerned about.

1:15 — Meet with 4 third grade students on production of /r/ and /s/.

1:30 — Meet with the librarian about a video she has on strategies for teaching students to become "researchers." (She thinks the information fits in with my philosophy of learning and wants my opinion.)

1:45 — Go into third grade classroom, where there are 10 language impaired/learning disabled students, meet with the resource teacher and implement a plan developed collaboratively with the classroom teacher on "poetry." Coach students to help them think of ideas. Use pictures to stimulate thinking. Discuss rhyming and word structure. Read some examples of poems and discuss descriptive language. Coach students who have decided to "work together" on how to have a "planning" conversation and how to "discuss" a topic.

2:45 — Go into fifth grade classroom. Coach my group of 5 language impaired students and 4 "normal" students on their social studies group project. (They are making a game to teach the other students key ideas from an assigned chapter.) The LI students need to develop logical questions and answers for the game, rules for the game, and construct the materials needed to play the game.

3:25 — Update student logs.

Thursday

7:45 — Review Team Meeting Schedule with school Principal.

8:00 — First Team Meeting of the day. In attendance are SLP, OT, school psychologist, special education teacher, classroom teacher, school principal, Chapter 1 coordinator, and parents. Academic concerns are discussed for a first grade student. After discussion of students strengths and weaknesses, referral for a language evaluation and occupational therapy evaluation is recommended. Further referrals will be made if needed after SLP and OT report findings.

8:45 — Second Team Meeting. Fifth grade student with severe behavior problems is discussed. Student is already on SLP's caseload. She reports difficulties with expressive and receptive language as well as frustration that student was not identified as learning disabled when evaluated by team as a second grade student. School principal, parents, and classroom teacher are also frustrated. Math skills appear to be a relative strength. Decision to reevaluate was made.

9:30 — Travel to preschool classroom.

9:45 — Observe students enrolled in morning preschool classroom and participate in planned classroom activities.

11:00 — Lunch with preschool teacher and her assistant to discuss individual preschool student's progress and needs.

12:00 — Observe students enrolled in afternoon preschool classroom and participate in planned classroom activities.

1:15 — Travel to elementary school.

1:45 — Evaluate student by conducting classroom observation, collecting narrative sample, reading a book together, collecting a written language sample, and administering selected standardized measures. Make note to set up a time to interview classroom teacher after school.

3:15 — Students dismissed. Classroom teacher says tomorrow at lunch would be a good interview time.

3:30 — Curriculum committee meeting in Media Center

Friday

7:45 — Set up for individual preschool therapy sessions which are conducted jointly with preschool teacher.

8:00 — First student arrives. Parent stays and watches the preschool teacher and me work with the student. We alternate leading and taking data. Student is very active, non-verbal, and benefits from team approach.

9:00 — Second student arrives. Preschool teacher begins with child while SLP talks with parent about the "choice board" that is proving very effective in the classroom during snack time and playtime. Parent will try to set one up at home. SLP joins preschool teacher for rest of session.

10:00 — Planning meeting with preschool teacher for next week, Update 2 students' goals and objectives. Discuss vocabulary selection for a student's AAC device.

10:45 — Travel to elementary school.

11:00 — Planning time with kindergarten teacher.

11:30 — Planning time with sixth grade teacher.

12:00 — Planning time with fourth grade teacher.

12:30 — Lunch (interview classroom teacher about student).

1:00 — Hearing screening.

1:15 — Planning time with first grade teachers.

2:00 — Planning time with second grade teacher.

2:30 — Planning time with third grade teacher.

3:00 — Planning time with fifth grade teacher.

3:15 — Student dismissal.

Under this schedule, a significant amount of time is devoted to planning and conferences. The teachers know that every other week they will be seeing Marilyn and together they will make their plans for the coming two-week period. The flexibility built into her new schedule made finding time to meet with teachers realistic. In addition, it made clear to everyone that planning and conferencing are priorities for Marilyn.

Summary

This account has made it sound as though Marilyn's entire focus during the first three or four years of her school practice was on changing her schedule. This was not the case, of course. Marilyn's students told her, through their struggles with academics, that they needed something different from her than they had had before. Remembering the vital role that language and communication play in the child's academic and social life, Marilyn felt compelled to find a way to unlock the system for the children. She was determined to make her intervention meaningful to the child's life, and for children in school that means the classroom and the peer group. With that premise in mind, Marilyn set herself the task of finding the best way to implement treatment within the context of the individual school environment. She found herself changing not only the place and the focus of her language intervention lessons, but also the concept of the role of language intervention for the child. Language intervention became much more than the traditional "pull the child out of the classroom and work on grammar or vocabulary and let the child figure out how it relates to the classroom." It became an integral part of the child's classroom life.

THE HUMAN SIDE OF CHANGE

Everyone who works with a child in the schools is an educator. The educators responsible for developing a language impaired student's Individual Educational Plan have a clear choice: They can decide through collaborative efforts to develop a program which provides consistency, predictability, emotional stability, and a sense of connection between communication proficiency and academic success. Or they can enroll the student in speech/language therapy, occupational therapy, physical therapy, special education class, and fourth grade as separate, unconnected entities. Choosing to collaborate means choosing to work together for the benefit of the student. It does not mean always having to agree. Compromise through cooperation should be the ideal. Collaboration cannot be forced on a group of educators by administrative fiat. Just as in every classroom there are a few students who would rather complete the science project alone, there are some teachers who would rather keep the doors to their classrooms and the pages of their plan books closed, and some speech-language pathologists who regard collaboration as an intrusion. The student, watching the children next to him work side by side to create an elaborate display and celebrate their success together at recess, may be motivated to work with a partner next time. So also, the teacher or speech-language pathologist hesitant to work with others to create a plan for helping a language impaired student succeed in History may simply need to watch it work somewhere else first. We must allow each other room to change at our individual rates.

Implementing Change

Statement of Principle: Although extremely adept at identifying those children in their classrooms with learning differences, classroom teachers have not been trained to identify those children for whom language impairment plays a significant role or to change the curriculum to meet these children's needs.

"Teambuilding" is the new buzzword in education, but the idea that two heads are better than one is not new. The question is how to begin. How do we interest a classroom teacher who historically has planned, taught, and problem solved autonomously, to work with a professional from another discipline? Marilyn realized that she needed a plan. She begin by outlining the foundations:

1. Literacy should be the goal for every student.
2. Language skills are intrinsic to literacy development.

3. Each student is entitled to an appropriate education in the least restrictive environment.
4. Children need predictability in their lives.

With these ideas as the basis for pursuing change, Marilyn seized any opportunity to share her ideas. She found herself talking frequently with two teachers who were very different, yet had several common traits.

Susan Jones was a fourth grade veteran teacher, very near retirement. She was well organized, a good listener, innovative, yet traditional in many ways. She impressed Marilyn with her observational skills and resourcefulness. She discussed teaching strategies with other teachers and always assumed that the child would learn if the teacher could understand individual strengths and weaknesses. She looked at each child as an individual, and considered any information that Marilyn provided about the language impaired children in her classroom to be both valuable and interesting. One day, as Marilyn and Susan talked at lunch, they discovered a mutual concern with vocabulary development in some of Susan's fourth grade students. Susan described how one language impaired child appeared able to decode the words in the History textbook, but was unable to interpret directions, define vocabulary, or answer comprehension questions at the end of each chapter. Marilyn asked to see the History text, and Susan found an extra teacher's edition for her. Marilyn then surprised Susan by saying that what she wanted was the student's edition, to find out exactly what the children were being confronted with. This gave Marilyn the chance to share her knowledge about text structure and specific vocabulary, and the difficulties language impaired children often experience with sequencing their ideas both in speaking and in writing.

The other teacher Marilyn began to work with was Ann Price, a special education resource teacher. Ann's basic teaching philosophy was based on the principles of Whole Language. She instructed students with learning disabilities, mild mental handicaps, and emotional handicaps in the areas of language arts and math, using a "pull-out" model. Ann was always looking for better ways to meet her students' needs. She was frustrated because she didn't have enough time to provide support for them in the content areas. Marilyn had pointed out to Ann that their caseloads almost entirely overlapped. Many of the children identified as language impaired were later diagnosed as learning disabled, mildly mentally handicapped, or emotionally handicapped. Ann had seen that, as her students increased their oral language skills, their thinking, reading, and writing skills improved as well. She was anxious to discover what areas she and Marilyn might collaborate on, so that they did not end up doing redundant programming for the children they worked with in common.

Marilyn had several language impaired children enrolled in Susan's classroom who were experiencing difficulty in the content areas. She discussed with Susan the idea of using the fourth grade History and Science textbooks as language therapy materials. Susan thought this was a great idea. "These kids really need help reading the textbooks," she said. Marilyn explained that she wouldn't be reading each chapter to the children. She described how she would teach them language based strategies for deciphering text, understanding directions, and storing new information.

At the same time, Ann and one of the kindergarten teachers with a language centered classroom and a Whole Language philosophy listened to Marilyn describe her experience with using children's literature as a context for language lessons. They shared their knowledge about children's authors and predictable books. The school librarian soon got word that Marilyn was using children's literature, and began pulling books from the shelf and putting them in her mailbox for review.

Marilyn had connected her goals for the language impaired students with what was happening in the students' classrooms. Although she was still pulling some of the children out for therapy, at least there was continuity at the ground level. Marilyn was using the curriculum as a basis for the language impaired students' programs.

SUMMARY

Every school speech-language pathologist will have an individual story to tell about setting up collaborative, classroom based intervention. Marilyn's story will be unique to her. We have told it here to give you some insight into the problems to be solved, the questions to be asked, and the creativity that will be demanded if you want to establish a program for language impaired children that is relevant to their education and focused on their needs as students in the classroom.

In describing how Marilyn set up her own practice, we have listed a number of principles we consider important for implementing collaborative classroom based intervention. A brief listing of these is presented below.

Principles

1. As speech-language pathologists, we must evaluate our current practices, challenge ourselves to develop progressive programs, and share

strategies for educating language impaired student through collaboration with school personnel and parents.

2. Oral and written language are the primary means by which a child demonstraes what has been learned within the school environment.

3. A speech-language pathologist should always be considered as part of the multidisciplinary team assembled to gather information about a student experiencing academic and/or social failure.

4. A collaborative classroom based model of language intervention must be implemented for all language impaired students if school success is a long range goal.

5. Although extremely adept at identifying those children in their classrooms with learning differences, classroom teachers have not been trained to identify those children for whom language plays a significant role nor have they been trained to change the curriculum to meet those children's needs.

We will turn our attention now to the two case studies, and see how Individual Educational Plans and goals might be established for Mitch and Jackie in the context of Marilyn's practice.

CLINICAL APPLICATIONS:
INTERVENTION WITH MITCH AND JACKIE

We will again allow you to listen in on another clinical brainstorming session similar to the ones presented in Chapter 1. Once again, our purpose is to present not only the thinking process involved in developing goals and objectives for each case, but also to share the process involved in clinical decision making. We hope that by reading our interaction you will again have the opportunity to visualize how collaboration inspires professional growth.

Clinical Brainstorming: Jackie

Debbie: Well, it looks as though the resource teacher's concerns about Jackie's language skills were justified. This evaluation revealed some truly significant language deficits which, I'm sure, are having an impact on Jackie's school success.

Rita: I think we have to do something quickly about Jackie's knowledge of narrative structure. If we can get some narrative framework established, she can then use that framework as a support for recall, for inferencing, and for reading comprehension.

Ann: It seems to me we want to do several things at once. We need to begin to work on the word finding problem, to help her use cues. We need to get the teacher involved in this cueing as soon as we can. Jackie is going to need help with finding the main idea in a text, and that is, of course, related to being able to tell what a story is about.

Debbie: We have to be sure to involve the teacher in the planning. We need to think about what we will need from her, and what can happen in the classroom.

Rita: OK, let's try to focus first on the work with narrative structure. I know we're going to want to work with trade books, maybe books the teacher has read or is reading to the class. Let's work with the teacher to choose some books.

Ann: We should choose a children's book with a strong problem/solution organization. [Problem/solution organization, and work with narrative structure, will be covered in Chapter 6.]

Debbie: Do we want to pick one part of narrative structure to focus Jackie on? Maybe on the beginning of a story?

Ann: I think we focus on story beginnings because they're the easiest for us. I'm not sure they're most useful for the child. The problem/solution structure is most useful for the child.

Debbie: Sort of the part you would use if you were telling what the story is about? It's true that when a child tells you what a story is about, they don't tell you the setting.

Ann: Exactly. Stories are about problems. This is where story structure starts to intersect with main idea .

Rita: And maybe after we read the book to Jackie, and talk with her about it, she can then write her own story based on the book. I like the idea of getting the child to compose as soon as possible, even if she dictates it and someone else writes it down for her.

Debbie: In my experience, it works better if the child dictates. Jackie is not good at the physical act of writing, and it takes a lot of time. I'd rather work with the language structures, and let the teacher work with letter formation and so on. But remember, Jackie will be able to take her "book" into the classroom to read to the teacher and to other children. The teacher is going to want to work on Jackie's writing using the same materials we're using. That will help her focus.

Rita: How "metalinguistic" do you feel comfortable getting? Do you want to say to Jackie something like "Stories are about problems and how people solve them?"

Ann: Yes. I might not do this with a younger child, but certainly with a child Jackie's age, you've got to be that clear about what you're doing.

Debbie: Maybe we could help her focus on problems and solutions by playing a matching game, putting problems on little slips of paper in one envelope, and solutions on little pieces of paper in another envelope, and having her draw a problem and then draw a solution, and talk about how well they fit. I'd like to have these problems all be classroom related—things like "Sally forgot to bring her homework to school." Let's get some ideas from the teacher.

Rita: I like this game, because we could model making up stories with the problem/solution pairs right there. And Jackie could make up her own stories.

Ann: I like the possibility for getting some humor into it. These random matches are likely to be pretty funny.

Debbie: I noticed in Jackie's account of her swimming lesson that the only cohesive devices she used were "then" and "and then." We need to work on this while she's making up stories. The teacher will be working on this in class as well. She calls them "transitions." [Work with cohesion is covered in Chapter 8.]

Ann: Jackie has some trouble with time concepts. Why don't we build in some use of "before" and "after" and also the "first, second, third" sequencing of events?

Rita: Good. Let's make a note to find some books with strong time sequencing in the events. These will provide us with a good base for working in these ideas.

Ann: Let's not forget that we want to carry this over to Jackie's comprehension of her textbooks. We need to have a bridge here.

Rita: I like the "idea map" approach. If we had a story about a polar bear, and we worked on an idea map about polar bears, where we put the polar bear in the middle of a circle, and then all around we put related ideas, like "snow" and "fish" and "hunting," we're engaging in the process Jackie will need to engage in to find a main idea. [Use of idea maps and other visual organizers is covered in Chapter 8.]

Debbie: Can we talk about that a little? I'm not sure I see the connection.

Ann: It goes back to the work of Baumann, who's done a book about how to teach main idea (Baumann, 1984). The basis of this is that what you're asking the child to do is categorize—to find a superordinate category for a group of connected ideas. You work the child up to this one step at a time, by working with single words, then with short phrases, then with sentences, and then with paragraphs. Children get the idea very quickly, because they are almost always successful finding a category, or a main idea, for groupings like "carrot, spinach, broccoli." If they say "food," we can get them down a level to "vegetable." It's a good process, and it's the sort of thing you're doing in reverse with an idea map. [Baumann's process is covered in detail in Chapter 8.]

Rita: Working a lot on this process should also help with Jackie's word finding. We'll be helping her to recognize the connections among various meanings in her store of concepts. The more work we do with storage and retrieval of these meanings, the better for Jackie.

Debbie: OK, let's see where we are. I'll meet with Jackie's teacher, and let her know that we'll be focusing on stories. I'll find out what she's been reading in class, and we'll talk about some books with strong time-based organization and good problem/solution structures. She might even want to pick a couple of these for the whole class to read. We'll read the book with Jackie, and talk about it. Jackie will write her own story based on the book. In addition, we'll focus her on problem/solution structure by playing our game, and making up some stories based on classroom problems. This will have the advantage of using her classroom script as support for her storying.

Ann: Right. And we'll also be doing some idea maps based on stories we read with Jackie, and we'll begin to work in some main idea teaching, so that by the end of the year, we'll be using her Social Studies and Science textbooks as materials for finding the main idea of a paragraph or chapter. And all along, we're going to have to focus on cues for this word finding problem. Alerting the teacher to the word finding difficulty, and working with the teacher on strategies to help Jackie in the classroom, should make a big difference here.

Developing the IEP

Let's now return Jackie's case to Marilyn, her speech-language pathologist, and observe the process by which goals and objectives were developed in collaboration with the teachers involved. Notice how the responsibility for providing a learning environment in which Jackie can be successful is shared by the speech-language pathologist, the special education teacher, and the classroom teacher. This is particularly important for a child like Jackie, who is both learning disabled and communication impaired.

Marilyn met with the resource teacher who had made the initial referral and the classroom teacher. She briefly discussed the results of the speech and language evaluation and suggested some goal areas. Both teachers indicated that they were unsure of what "word finding" difficulties involved. Marilyn defined the term for them and gave several examples using data collected from her observation of Jackie in the classroom. As the concept became clear to them, they each recalled several situations in which Jackie had experienced difficulty retrieving familiar information. Marilyn continued by reporting that Jackie demonstrated weaknesses in narrative skills, inferencing abilities, and auditory memory for language. Both teachers made comments which supported Marilyn's findings, so she developed some specific goals and objectives for recommendation at the Case Conference. They were as follows:

Goal: Jackie will demonstrate use of cognitive schemata (mental frameworks) for comprehending large units of text (stories) important for school success.

> **Objective:** Jackie will become familiar with story structure and the language of stories by participating in read-aloud sessions on a daily basis.
> **Objective:** Jackie will identify and relate problem(s) and solution(s) within the context of simple stories.
> **Objective:** Jackie will identify and relate the main idea of a story.

Objective: Jackie will retell complete episodes within a story using story language.

Goal: Jackie will increase her use of strategies to compensate for word-finding problems.

Objective: Jackie will verbally indicate that she is having word-finding problems by saying something like, "I know what it is but I can't think of it right now."
Objective: Jackie will use cues provided by the teacher(s) and parent to formulate a response.
Objective: Jackie will use self-cuing strategies to formulate a response.
Objective: Jackie will employ rehearsal strategies for new and familiar vocabulary.

Goal: Jackie will develop strategies for inferencing to increase comprehension and memory for information read or heard.

Objective: Jackie will demonstrate use of logical categories for organizing personal experiences.
Objective: Jackie will indicate when her personal experiences are limited for a given topic.
Objective: Jackie will respond to cues to recall relevant personal experiences within the context of a shared book experience.

During Jackie's case conference, the goals and objectives were approved. Marilyn explained to the parent that she and the teachers would be working together with Jackie toward completion of the goals and objectives. In addition, she wrote on the IEP under the "Method of Evaluation" section that:

Progress towards completion of these goals and objectives will be determined by those responsible for implementation of the IEP through a review of student portfolio, conferences, and collaborative consultation.

Next, a decision was needed regarding the "least restrictive environment" for Jackie, to meet the goals and objectives. Marilyn explained that she wanted to work with Jackie using a classroom based approach to intervention. In other words, she would meet with Jackie's teacher every couple of weeks, and gather information about what part of the curriculum was currently being presented in the classroom. Jackie's classroom teacher added, "There might be times when having the special education resource teacher or Marilyn come into the classroom to coach Jackie would be beneficial." The Case Conference Committee decided that a combination of pull-out and inclusive programming would be the least restrictive environment for Jackie to reach her goals and objectives.

> The Individuals With Disabilities Education Act (IDEA) is a Federal law which guarantees four rights and two protections for each child with a disability and his/her parent. One of these is an education within the least restrictive environment, which means that students with disabilities are to be educated as much as possible with students who have no disabilities, with the appropriate amount of time being determined on an individual basis.

The next questions asked related to intervention for word finding. The principal, who was chairing the conference, asked for some examples of strategies to use when Jackie came into the school office to deliver a message. Marilyn explained that it is impossible to predict with any certainty when a child will have a word finding problem. She said, "We want Jackie to come to understand the difficulty that she has and to learn to compensate for it. In order to do this it is important that we all collaborate and provide her with the support and encouragement she needs." Marilyn reviewed the strategies outlined in the objectives and gave examples of each. She explained that it was important to give Jackie time to formulate what she wanted to say, and that sometimes it might help to give her either/or choices to help her retrieve words. Then she added, "It is important that we share with one another our observations about which strategies work best for Jackie and communicate that information to everyone else in her environment."

Clinical Brainstorming: Mitch

Debbie: Well, the results of the language evaluation have really given us some good information for developing a plan for this year. I'm glad Mitch is in a classroom with a teacher who has a Whole Language philosophy. Mitch needs to have lots of opportunities to see how oral and written language are connected before phonics can make much sense to him.

Rita: Eventually, he will need to develop some basic phonological awareness. Using context clues to decode words won't be easy for Mitch either. After all, that involves inferencing, which we know he has trouble with.

Debbie: That's true. We'll need to make developing metalinguistic skills a goal for him.

Ann: Maybe we can tap into his strengths with visual memory and visual sequencing noted by the school psychologist. We could probably develop his narrative skills at the same time.

Rita: That would be great. And whatever strategies we develop must be shared with the classroom teacher and parents. I know they are both frustrated because Mitch didn't qualify for services as a learning disabled student.

Debbie: They need to know that his classification as communication impaired doesn't mean he'll get no help with learning. I learned a strategy from a special education resource teacher that we might be able to adapt for Mitch. We know from our testing that he has trouble with recounting events logically, right?

Ann: Right. He seems to have real difficulty attaching language to his scripts.

Debbie: Well, the resource teacher has kids develop a "word box." A child tells her a word that he wants to learn to read, she writes it down on an index card, and the child puts it in a "word box." Because the word has meaning to the child he can usually remember it when asked to read it. We could have Mitch pick a familiar routine, and help him develop a script for it. Then we could write it down and put key words on index cards. He could learn to read the card and use it as a cue to recount the event logically.

Ann: That would be something we could give the classroom teacher to do also as part of Mitch's reading program. I was also thinking about using books with predictable plots with Mitch. His knowledge of episode structure is so weak at this point.

Rita: I'm concerned about his vocabulary development and his ability to elaborate his meanings. We should work on eliciting descriptions and every time he gives us a description, we ask for more. A bigger vocabulary of descriptive words will help here, but just practicing doing it will help as well. Maybe we could start using some primitive "idea maps" with him to help him see how much there is to say about some of his topics.

Ann: We should make sure that we find out what themes they'll be studying in the classroom during our planning time with his teacher.

Debbie: I know that she will be using the mapping strategy a lot in the classroom. That fits right into the Whole Language philosophy. Whenever a discussion takes place someone is either making a list on chart paper or making an idea map on the overhead projector.

Rita: It sounds like there will be plenty of good opportunities to work directly within the classroom with Mitch as a coach.

Debbie: I'm a little worried about his reticence in the classroom. The evaluation results and his school history suggest problems with conversation. Coaching will help, but we're not in the classroom all the time, and the teacher has a whole class to manage.

Rita: Maybe the teacher could have Mitch sit near a more verbal child so that he always has a peer model. Of course, it would be important that the verbal child didn't take over and talk for Mitch.

Ann: Maybe he could be taught some scripts for playing games with fairly simple rules. We could work with Mitch during recess one day and he could ask a friend to play. That would put him in the talking role.

Rita: What do you think about the CELF-R results? I'm concerned about the score on the Following Directions subtest.

Debbie: The teacher and his parents agreed that they see it as a weakness too. At the initial referral meeting they described him as often being confused.

Ann: I'd like to see the teacher encourage him to make lists to keep track of what he needs to do. We could work with him on this and help him develop some strategies for making sure he follows his list.

Debbie: It also uses his strength in the visual modality again. It really should be a logical thing for him to do in the classroom because the Whole Language philosophy stresses using oral and written language meaningfully as a crucial part of becoming literate.

Rita: Well, it sounds like we are ready to develop some goals and objectives. Let's set up a meeting with his classroom teacher and determine a date for the case conference.

We will now return Mitch to his speech-language pathologist, Marilyn, as she collaborates with his classroom teacher. Each of them has an important role to play in the development of his Individual Education Plan.

Developing Mitch's IEP

Marilyn met with Mitch's classroom teacher. She discussed briefly the results of the evaluation, and the fact that Mitch would be recommended for continuation in language therapy at the upcoming case conference. Marilyn then shared a list of goal areas with the teacher and asked her to suggest a few to target with Mitch. With the teacher's suggestions in mind and the information from the speech and language evaluation, Marilyn developed some specific goals and objectives to be recommended at the case conference. These were as follows:

Goal: Mitch will follow oral and written directions within the school setting.

> **Objective:** Mitch will use language to relate the meaning of the phrase "follow the directions" within the context of classroom activities.
> **Objective:** Mitch will use language to relate the meaning of vocabulary frequently associated with oral and written direction.
> **Objective:** Mitch will use reauditorization skills when given a two-step direction within the context of a school routine or learning activity.
> **Objective:** Given the materials to complete an assignment, Mitch will use general knowledge gained from past experiences to complete the task independently.

Goal: Mitch will develop metalinguistic skills.

Objective: Mitch will demonstrate comprehension of the terms "letter," "word," and "story" by supplying a logical definition and examples of each.
Objective: Mitch will accurately count the number of words in a given sentence and the number of letters in a given word consistently.
Objective: Given a word, Mitch will locate the first and last letters consistently.

Goal: Mitch will use narratives to demonstrate cognitive schemata (mental frameworks) for a variety of concepts, actions, and events important for school success.

Objective: Mitch will relate organized, coherent accounts of routine events using key words such as "first," "next," "then," and "last."
Objective: Mitch will relate organized, coherent, plans for events (eventcasts).
Objective: Mitch will become familiar with story structure and the language of stories by participating in read-aloud sessions daily.

Goal: Mitch will converse appropriately about a variety of topics by integrating world knowledge, linguistic knowledge, and knowledge of how to negotiate meanings.

Objective: Mitch will develop strategies for determining what information the conversational partner needs to know.
Objective: Mitch will demonstrate appropriate topic maintenance strategies by maintaining a topic of interest for at least three conversational turns.

At the case conference the goals and objectives were approved. The implementors of the IEP were determined by the case conference committee to be the speech-language pathologist and the classroom teacher.

A commitment to a collaborative model of intervention allows any number of school personnel to be designated as implementors of a student's Individual Education Plan.

The need for classroom modifications was also discussed at the case conference and documented on Mitch's IEP. The need for visual support and a holistic approach to teaching reading were discussed. The classroom teacher explained that she incorporates a significant amount of visual support into her classroom environment already by writing the daily schedule on the chalkboard. Marilyn suggested numbering the day's events sequentially. The classroom teacher said she could make that Mitch's "job" each day, and everyone agreed that was a good idea.

Marilyn and Mitch's teacher decided to work together on developing his metalinguistic skills, and agreed he should have access to predictable books that tied into the class's current thematic unit of study for reading instruction. Together, they also developed a few sequenced activities for the classroom which Mitch would be asked to describe his small group therapy sessions.

SUMMARY

Our goal in this chapter has been to introduce you to the nature of a collaboratiave, curriculum based intervention model. Our hope is that you will come away from it with the realization that it is an infinitely flexible model, within which the individual needs of a variety of children might be met. It does not mean that a child will never have individual work outside the classroom. It does mean that what a child does in the time away from the classroom will be directly related to what is happening in the classroom. It also does not mean that the speech-language pathologist becomes a tutor, teaching the same content as the classroom teacher. It does mean that the speech-language pathologist works with language impaired children to help them develop strategies that will allow them to make classroom content meaningful. These strategies are not content specific, but are instead generalizable across content areas. Finally, as Marilyn, our school speech-language pathologist said, "The greatest benefit of this practice model is that at last I feel like a real educator. I'm not a fringe person who interrupts the child's education. I am a part of what this child gets from school, and the teacher, the parents, and the child know this." This is the way we'd like every school practitioner to feel.

C H A P T E R 3

The Not-So-Simple Art
of Conversation

The purpose of this chapter is to provide you with a framework for talking about conversation, and for understanding the sorts of difficulties language impaired children have with conversation. The variables we use to analyze children's conversations will be defined and discussed, followed by a case study of one child whose conversational abilities were the focus for intervention.

TALKING ABOUT CONVERSING

What does it take to engage in conversations? On the face of it, nothing seems to be more simple or more natural for human beings to do than to talk with one another. Two-year-olds can do it, and so can some people whose speech abilities are so impaired that they must use an augmentative system to convey their messages. Much of the research on the development of communication skills has corroborated this picture of conversation as a fairly easy activity. Generally, researchers have analyzed children's conversations by examining them turn by turn, looking at such factors as relevant turntaking, topic setting and maintenance, and perhaps at repairing of conversational breakdowns. The typical approach to this task is to concentrate on only one variable at a time, such as turn-taking, while ignoring the rest, as if the separate categories were immune to one another's influence. Using this model, researchers have found that while language impaired children do converse, their turns are shorter and linguistically less complex than those of their peers, they can speak on topic, although they seldom initiate topics themselves, and they have some limited ability to repair conversational breakdowns (Rice, Sell, & Hadley, 1991; Rosinski-McClendon & Newhoff, 1987; Craig & Gallagher, 1986; Snyder, 1984; Fey & Leonard, 1983; Brinton & Fujiki, 1982; Gallagher & Darnton, 1978). This single-variable approach to conversation (Kellerman, Broetzmann, Lim, & Kitao, 1989) has given rise to an almost exclusively linguistic explanation for the differences found between conversations of language normal and language impaired children. That is, language impaired children are supposed to be less able to understand and construct sentences because of their limited knowledge of syntax and phonology, and consequently are less mature conversationalists.

This explanation, while intuitively appealing, tells us little about language impaired children's conversations that we did not already know, and it may even mislead us in a critical respect: such explanations ignore the fact that older language impaired children may, in fact, not have noticeable impairments of either phonology or syntax, and yet are often poor conversationalists. In addition, linguistically based explanations ignore the fact that, as Bruner (1983) points out, "the rules of language use are only lightly specified by the rules of grammar" (p.119). Bruner goes on to say that well-formed utterances are not necessarily either appropriate or effective, and by extension, we might also say that ill-formed utterances are not necessarily inappropriate or ineffective. The point here is that learning syntax and phonology does not necessarily make a child an adept conversationalist. Any of us who have ever learned a second language in the classroom, doing well on all the grammar tests, and then tried to converse in the language with native speakers will know this.

Those who work with language impaired children on a daily basis find the linear, linguistically based approach reflected in most research findings frustrating, and often say "There's something weird about this child's interactions—and it's more than not knowing grammar." This difference between language competence and language use is especially visible once a language impaired child has developed sufficient expressive syntax to be able to construct four to five word utterances. A description of the child's syntactic or lexical abilities is not likely to be terribly revealing to anyone attempting to describe the child's problems with communication. For many such children of school age, tests of receptive syntax indicate normal performance, and tests of expressive syntax show only slight delays, despite the claims by teachers, parents, and speech/language pathologists that there is something "wrong" with the child's "language." Our clinical frustrations are reflected by the scarcity of research literature on the topic. We know a great deal about the linguistic performance of those children we call "language impaired," but we have little data and fewer theoretical explanations related to how these children employ their linguistic competence in the service of communication.

Perhaps we can't see what is wrong with these children because we assume conversations are simple events. We can begin to move beyond this assumption by returning to our initial question: What does it take to engage in conversation? What sorts of abilities do normal conversationalists have which might be lacking in the person who is perceived as being an impaired conversationalist? To address this question, we must recognize that conversation is not simply a sort of verbal tennis game in which two people bat a message back and forth, each taking a turn as the sender or the receiver. A successful conversation is in fact an enormously complex undertaking, in which the participants negotiate not only the meanings for individual utterances, but also the contextual framework in which the utterances are to be interpreted and judged for appropriateness. As Fredriksen (1981) expresses it:

> A participant must, at the opening of a conversation make a preliminary interpretation of the situation and other participants' talk, construct an appropriate contextual frame to represent the speech event as it has developed thus far, produce conversational acts that at the same time satisfy local conversational constraints and communicate an intended meaning within the frame, and reinterpret the frame as the interaction develops and the activity changes or becomes more completely negotiated (p. 310).

When Fredricksen talks about conversational **frameworks**, he is talking about the acts the conversationalists are engaged in; that is, whether a conversation is a dispute, a problem-solving session, a recounting of a past event, etc. This is not the same as the conversational **topic**. A dispute **framework** might be about the topic of money, or who lost the car keys. An event recounting might be about the topic of a tragic car accident or a vacation trip. We are perhaps more accustomed to thinking about conversations in terms of their topics, but the conversational framework will have its own set of constraints and conventions, and as frameworks shift in the course of a conversation, the participants must **negotiate meaning** just as they do when topics shift.

Just what is it we know when we know about conversational frameworks? We know both what kinds of things we can do with words, and how to do those things. We know how to tell a story, how to gossip, how to have an argument, how to tell a joke, how to criticize, how to establish solidarity with a group, how to recount experience, and on and on. Conversational frameworks are the macrostructures we use for organizing and making sense of our talk with other people. Fredricksen (1981) contends that it is conversational frameworks which make possible inferences about conversational meaning. Our knowledge of the conventions of frameworks makes it possible to interpret not only the literal meaning of the words we hear, but also all the "between the lines" meaning that goes to make up the whole of the conversational message. For example, imagine that you and your favorite cousin are reminiscing about your shared childhoods at a family reunion. Recalling several events the two of you shared, your cousin laughs and says, "You have perfected the art of being late. You were probably even born late." Now imagine that your supervisor is evaluating your recent job performance. She says, "You have perfected the art of being late. You were probably even born late." The words are the same, but there is a world of difference in the meanings being conveyed. We are able to appreciate these meanings in part because we understand the conventions of the two frameworks within which the utterance is occurring. Now imagine a language impaired first grade girl, eager to be accepted into a peer group at school. The children in the class are playing the familiar "boys against the girls" game of tag and capture at recess. The girls have momentarily huddled together to verbally attack the boys, to talk about how mean and rude and rough they are. This is talk intended to build solidarity among the group of girls. It is in many ways formulaic and full of hyperbole, and to participate in it demands that one be able to make an utterance that restates the basic meaning of "boys are horrible," either by telling about some specific instance of awful behavior, or by generalizing from such an instance. The language impaired child must be able to figure out not only how to construct a phonologically and syntactically adequate proposition, but also exactly what sort of meaning is appropriate to this conversational event and when it should be inserted into the ongoing stream. This is exceptionally demanding on-line processing, and the need for it may account for many more of the language impaired child's conversational problems than we have realized.

Consider the following conversation between two five-year-olds in their kindergarten classroom as an example of how frameworks shift and meanings get negotiated in the course of even a brief conversation:

1. **A.** What are you doing?
2. **B.** Cutting this picture.

3. **A.** Who said you could?
4. **B.** Miss Sandy, and besides, I don't have to ask.
5. **A.** You do too have to ask, because you can't use the scissors.
6. **B.** I, I have scissors myself and I don't have to ask for any.
7. **A.** Well, if you make a mess you're going to have to stay in at juice time and then you won't have any snack.
8. **B.** You're not the teacher. Bossy pants.
9. **A.** I am not bossy pants. You're not very nice.
10. **B.** You're the one that's not nice, bossy pants.
11. **A.** I'm telling.
12. **B.** Baby bossy pants.

A simple conversational analysis might examine the utterance pairs 1/2, 3/4, etc. to determine whether the turns taken by the two children were related, and if so, how. A bit more complicated analysis would examine larger units of the conversation than these utterance pairs, with the goal of finding topic initiations and shifts. Fredriksen (1981) is proposing that we go a step beyond this in abstraction, and look at the contextual frames the participants are establishing, to understand how meaning is communicated within the frame, and how the frame is dynamically renegotiated. With this latter goal in mind, we can note that the conversational opening provided by child A is a typical opening salvo used by children in task related interactions, and as such it sets only a general topic within a framework of "Let's talk". By labeling his task, child B both agrees to participate in this framework and adds to the framework by narrowing the topic. Child A then narrows the context and defines the framework. This is not going to be a conversation about cutting pictures. We are now engaged in a **dispute** (the contextual frame) about **authority** (the conversational topic). Note that child B implicitly agrees to this framework by answering A's question and issuing a challenge of his own. The dispute framework continues through utterance #6, along fairly conventional lines. It is clear that both children know how to engage in a verbal dispute. Then suddenly, in utterance #7, two things happen. Child A signals a topic shift with the word "well," and also moves to shift the framework. She is no longer engaged in a dispute about authority, she has assumed authority and opens the way for a discussion of penalties. Child B refuses both the topic shift and the new framework, but he does so implicitly by saying "You're not the teacher." This utterance indicates that he has (1) understood that A is taking on the teacher's role, and (2) not agreed to allow A to be the teacher in this situation. His utterance carries a multitude of meanings, from "I don't have to listen to you" to "I'm getting tired of this interaction." Furthermore, he issues another challenge, in effect saying "And not only are you not the teacher, you're a bossy pants." With this utterance, he moves to continue the previous dispute framework. Child A at this point gives over control of the interaction to B, by focusing on the name-calling rather than on her previous topic, and the conversation rapidly degenerates into a routine familiar to any teacher or parent. All of this negotiated meaning takes place, of course, in a larger context (the classroom) which allows both children to make some inferences about asking and giving permission and acceptable reasons for behavior, along with roles appropriate to each other within this context. Thinking about this conversation from the perspective of how the children use the frames, we can see that both of them know the conventions for having a dispute. They know what you do in a conversational turn if you're having a dispute. They know how to interpret what the other person does. They know how to move to change the framework, and how to reject such a move. This knowledge accounts in large part for the smoothness of the turntaking and the absence of conversational breakdown. At the same time, another kind of knowledge also underlies the conversation. Without a shared "classroom" schema, it is unlikely that this conversation could have proceeded as it did. Both children know that you have to ask permission for some things (including, apparently, using the scissors), that the permission must be granted by a person in authority, and that this authority also has the right to assign consequences to certain forbidden actions. None of this shared knowledge is made explicit in the conversation, but it is clear that without it, many of the individual utterances would be nonsense. The children in this example are assuming some shared information, and are basing their conversational meanings on this shared information and on their framework knowledge, using it to construct the new meanings of the conversation.

TAKING ANOTHER LOOK AT CONVERSATIONAL MEANING

The example above, and our analysis of it, suggests that focusing on meanings in conversations will necessitate our talking about two kinds of meaning: the meaning we assume, and the meaning we negotiate. Assumed meaning is sometimes referred to as **presuppositional meaning.** Presuppositional meaning involves a special kind of knowledge, which some people have called "social" knowledge. When we interact with other people, we are constantly adjusting the level of information we convey, in terms of what we believe the other person already knows, or doesn't know, about the topic. Our goal, of course, is to give exactly the right kind and amount of information—not too little, not too much. The two children in the example conversation above didn't have to explain to each other that using scissors without permission was not allowed in the classroom. Each of them knew this, and each of them assumed the other's knowledge of the rule. In contrast to this successful presupposing, young children often assume that everyone they talk to knows everything they know, so they may fail to give enough information for their listeners to interpret what they are saying. Older children also sometimes make this mistake, as the following conversation between a 10 year old boy and his teacher shows:

[F. is describing a movie he watched]

F: Well, see, this guy was watching these men, and he wasn't supposed to, and then this one guy, he saw him, and they started to chase him, and he was hiding behind this thing, and then he jumped over it and, you know, he shot at him.

T: Wait, I'm confused. Who jumped, and who got shot?

F: The spy man, he jumped over this big thing he was hiding behind and the bad guy shot him. And my favorite part was when they went down this street, you know, and they were bumping into each other, and these, like little pieces of fire were coming off, you know.

T: I'm confused again. Who was going down the street? And why were they bumping into each other?

F: The two cars, where the bad guys were chasing the other guy, and they kept bumping into him to try to push him off the road, and it was making fire, and they thought maybe the gas tank would explode.

As we can see from this exchange, F. consistently talks about the movie in terms which would be quite comprehensible if his teacher had been watching it with him, so that she shared all his knowledge about it. His failure to make his meaning clear was not due to a linguistic inability to do so. We can see by his responses to the teacher's questions that he could clarify when she let him know that he needed to. The problem was, it didn't seem to occur to him to do so until he was prompted. Many language impaired children, however, have a dual problem with presuppositional meaning. First, they, like F., don't make proper presuppositions. They seem to be unaware of the necessity to figure out what the listener probably knows or doesn't know about the topic. And second, they are not good at referential communication even when they are certain that the listener has no relevant information. Conversations with language impaired children are often a series of confusions for listeners because of their problems with presuppositional meaning.

Another relevant meaning related concept is negotiated meaning. The idea that what people are doing in a conversation is negotiating meaning is not a new one, of course. Gordon Wells (1981), among others, has discussed this concept at length. What is implied here is that what we say in a conversation with another person involves more than the meaning we started with in our own mind. It also involves the meaning the other person constructs based on our words, and our response to that meaning. In the conversation that follows, a mother and her 6 year old daughter negotiate a meaning connected with birthdays and aging which is unlike the meaning either of them had when they started the conversation.

M: What should we do for grandma's birthday?
D: When is it?
M: It's this coming Saturday.
D: How old will she be?
M: She'll be 75. That's a very special birthday.
D: That's pretty old.
M: Yes, although lots of people live to be older than that.
D: Will grandma get a lot older?
M: Well, we certainly hope so. She's healthy, and she takes good care of herself.
D: How old are you, mom?
M: I'm 40, dear.
D: Is that very old?
M: No, not at all. I have 35 more years before I'm as old as grandma. By the time I'm grandma's age, you'll be as old as I am now.
D: That's a long, long, long time. How old will you get to be?
M: You mean before I die?
D: Yeah.
M: Oh, about a hundred, I expect.
D: And will grandma get to be a hundred?
M: Well, she certainly might, if she keeps on like she is now.
D: So nobody is going to die for a long time.
M: Well, we hope not.

This is what is meant by negotiating meaning, and the ability to negotiate meaning is one of the main differences between conversations and lectures or sermons. When only one person talks, without response by others, there is no possibility to have multiple meanings made evident. However, as soon as two (or more) people can talk and respond to each other, multiple meanings are made evident, and if understanding is to occur, these multiple meanings must become a single negotiated meaning. Successful negotiation demands that the conversationalists stay within the bounds of the framework and the topic until the meanings associated with them have been made clear. It also demands that framework or topic changes must be clearly marked, so that joint meanings can continue to be negotiated. An unmarked topic or framework shift will preclude the possibility of negotiated meanings altogether. The kinds of subtle topic shadings and cohesive ties that we see in the example above between the 6 year old and her mother are beyond many language impaired children. To achieve negotiated meanings in a conversation, they must depend heavily on contextual support and the scaffolding of other participants. One appropriate goal for such children must involve learning some strategies to give them access to the negotiation of meanings.

Fredricksen's focus on the need for a meaning based approach to analyzing what is going on in conversations promises a rich explanation for what happens in conversation and also for what happens when conversations break down. By attending to conversational frameworks and the meanings we negotiate within them, we can often clarify conversational moves that traditional linear approaches do not discover (Kellerman et al., 1989), and we can gain a new perspective for describing the sorts of conversational problems language impaired children are having.

Conversation and Language Impaired Children

This focus on meaning suggests that there is one important question we will confront when we consider the special case of a language impaired child as a conversationalist: what kinds of framework and real-world and social knowledge can this child bring to bear in a conversation? We know that children must be able to understand the frameworks they are working within in order to construct utterances appropriate to those frameworks. For example, part of a child's conversational competence involves the knowledge that a threat is not an appropriate move in a problem solving discussion, and that making a threat is likely to result at the very least in a framework shift. Children learn this sort of thing by virtue of their participation in conversations. Some of this knowledge will result from suffering the consequences of framework violations, and some of it will result from direct instruction. Language impaired children may have many problems with framework knowledge, not least among them problems with initiating participation in them to begin with. Children must also have sufficient real-world knowledge and social knowledge about other people to enable them to work within the web of shared implicit knowledge that results in appropriate presuppositions in conversation. Language impaired children seem to have sometimes overwhelming difficulties with presupposition, and they may alternate between telling their listeners too much detail and not telling enough to make their references clear.

The question we always come down to as clinicians is: Why can't language impaired children engage in the dynamic renegotiation of contexts and messages? What limitations prohibit them from such activities? Can language impaired children's failures as conversationalists best be explained as indicating a lack of knowledge, a lack of on-line processing using the knowledge, or a lack of on-line translation into sentences of what has been processed? A child who does not engage in conversation in an appropriate way may simply not have enough knowledge, about frameworks or conversational conventions, to participate. Alternatively, a child may not be able to keep up in a conversation because things are happening too fast. If a child needs more than the normal amount of time to process spoken language or to encode meaning, conversing at a normal rate will be impossible. Finally, a child might fail as a conversationalist because of a processing overload. The demands of forming sentences, comprehending the sentences of others, discerning the topic and the framework, negotiating meaning to stay within topic and framework, making appropriate presuppositions based on shared knowledge, etc., may simply overwhelm the child's resources, resulting in the necessity to respond to some or all of these demands in less complex ways.

Language impaired children are not all alike. Regardless of how useful it might be to have one explanation for conversational failure which could be attached to every child, it is not possible to choose one of the explanations listed above and declare that this is the reason all language impaired children have problems with conversation. A given child's difficulties may be attributed to any one, or any combination of, these explanations. Furthermore, while knowing the underlying cause of a child's difficulty may affect our approach to intervention with that child (For example, do we need to slow down the input to the child? Do we need to teach the child some of the underlying knowledge? Do we need to reduce the processing demands?), we still need to know where in a conversation the child is having the most difficulty. In attempting to decide where to intervene, it seems most profitable to look at conversation as a network of negotiated meanings, and to learn to identify those points in the conversation which are taxing the child. We can then begin to focus on strategies to help with these.

SUMMARY

Conversation is a complex activity. Add to this the fact that conversationalists cannot think of one piece of the conversation at a time, but must do everything at once, and the language impaired child's difficulties become more understandable. The facility with which normal speakers engage in conversation is almost certainly a result of our overlearning of both linguistic rules and pragmatic conventions—we say that these have been overlearned because they no longer demand conscious thought as we employ them. The negotiation of framework, topic, and meaning within even a brief conversation demands controlled attention and memory. For most children, the scaffolding of familiar event representations and frameworks facilitates and supports this controlled processing. For language impaired children, however, this picture is likely to be very different. Linguistic and pragmatic rules may not be fully learned, and controlled, conscious processing is demanded when the child employs these. Conversational negotiation places additional demands on resources, and the ability to depend on shared event representations and framework knowledge may be lacking as well. Given this, it is not so surprising that many language impaired children are poor conversationalists.

ANALYZING A CHILD'S CONVERSATION: GEORGE

What follows is a case study and our analysis of the child's conversational abilities. The analysis system we use is different from those usually seen in the research literature. We have chosen it both for its clinical utility and for its fit with the meaning based approach to conversation reflected so far in this chapter. The next chapter will contain our intervention plan, based on this analysis.

George was 11 years old when he was brought to the attention of the school speech-language pathologist. He had attended school in another district for three years, and had been classified as emotionally handicapped by the school psychologist in that system. For the last year, he had been home schooled by his mother, but she had decided that this was not a good solution for him. She was ready to put him back in school, but she was adamant that she wanted him in a regular classroom. She did not believe he was emotionally handicapped, although she admitted that he had some problems. In particular, she expressed concern that he seemed not to have any friends among his peers. She also reported that she was worried about him because, as she said, "When we go out to the mall, or anywhere like that, he walks up to perfect strangers and starts conversations with them. I've told him over and over that this is dangerous, but he keeps doing it."

George was placed in a regular fourth grade classroom, and we began observation during the first week of school. He was fairly well behaved in the classroom, in that he did not cause any disturbances, but he frequently appeared to be "tuning out." He would stare into space, with a vacant look on his face. When he did this, he would respond immediately when the teacher called his name. At recess, he did not attempt to interact with the other children. He stayed with the teacher on duty, and engaged in long, rambling monologues. His approach to the teacher was always in terms of a well learned routine: he would walk up, and in a cheerful tone, say "Hi. My name is George. How are you today?" When the teacher replied "Fine. How are you?" as each one did in some form or other, George would immediately begin to talk. His conversation seldom dealt with the immediate context, and almost inevitably resulted in the teacher looking confused and beginning to ask him clarifying questions. When George was put into a small work group in the classroom, and asked to help design a plan for an Indian village, he was largely silent. When asked direct questions by another child, such as "What do you think, George, should we have one river or two?" he would frequently answer as though he had not heard the question. The other children would roll their eyes and pretend not to have heard him. After he had been in the classroom for two weeks, his teacher spoke with the speech-language pathologist. "I think he doesn't understand questions," she said. "He seems to know that an answer is called for, but he rarely gives an answer that is even in the ballpark. And then, every once in awhile, he seems to tune in and give you the right answer. Mostly, I'd say, he doesn't make any difference between 'how' and 'why' and 'when'." We decided to videotape George interacting with the school speech language pathologist, to get a conversational sample we could use for analysis. That sample is given below.

George and S. (the SLP) are seated together at a table in a small room. The video camera, operated by another adult, is across the table from them. The notation ... indicates a pause of at least 3 seconds.

1. **S:** I'd like for you to tell me what your favorite TV program is.
2. **G:** Ah, ah, Silver Spoons.
3. **S:** Silver Spoons?
4. **G:** Uh huh.

 5. **S:** Can you tell me what happens on that program?
 6. **G:** Yeah, you spill some ink.
 7. **S:** On the TV show?
 8. **G:** Uh huh.
 9. **S:** Then what happens?
10. **G:** Pour a glass of water on the floor.
11. **S:** Did that happen on TV?
12. **G:** Yeah.
13. **S:** Can you tell me another part?
14. **G:** [No reponse. Makes humming sounds]
15. **S:** Are there kids on that show?
16. **G:** What?
17. **S:** Silver Spoons. Are there kids on that show?
18. **G:** Uh huh.
19. **S:** What do they do?
20. **G:** Watch TV.
21. **S:** Uh huh.
22. **G:** [Looks at camera operator.] What's your name?
23. **K:** Kim.
24. **G:** Kim, hi.
25. **K:** Hi, George.
26. **G:** Uh, nice to meet you.
27. **K:** Nice to meet you too.
28. **S:** Let's see what I've got in here [takes out a small robot]. This is a transformer, George. [Twists the robot's head] Look what that did.
29. **G:** I ask the family ... what, what they're going to have ... bacon.
30. **S:** What family?
31. **G:** Marianne next door.
32. **S:** Oh, you asked the family next door what they were going to have?
33. **G:** You ever met her?
34. **S:** No, I don't know Marianne. She's your neighbor?
35. **G:** Uh huh.
36. **S:** And she's going to have bacon for dinner or breakfast?
37. **G:** Bacon.
38. **S:** Is she gonna have bacon for breakfast?
39. **G:** Uh huh. Put eggs in it and dip in it.
40. **S:** Uh huh.
41. **G:** Then ... twist it a little bit with a fork. If you get right close to you the bacon will, might, will pop on you.
42. **S:** Then what would happen?
43. **G:** You'll put cold water.
44. **S:** Uh huh. It'll burn you?
45. **G:** Uh huh.
46. **S:** And then you put cold water on the burn, right?
47. **G:** Right.

48. **S:** Did you ever make bacon, George?
49. **G:** Uh huh.
50. **S:** At your house?
51. **G:** Yeah.
52. **S:** Do you ever cook anything else? What else do you cook?
53. **G:** [overlapping with last question] Eggs.
54. **S:** Uh huh.
55. **G:** I used to cry for eggs when I was little.
56. **S:** You liked them a lot, huh?
57. **G:** Yeah.
58. **S:** How do you make eggs?
59. **G:** Put butter ... then put those away, melts, dip an egg and crack it. Put it in wastebastik, ket. Put it up and push it up a little bit like the rest of the eggs. You eat the ... you cook them then you put it on your plate then you eat them. That's how you cook eggs.
60. **S:** Yeah. That's how you cook them. Do you like robots, George?
61. **G:** Yeah, I love chili.
62. **S:** Uh huh. Do you cook chili too?
63. **G:** Uh huh. Macaroni.
64. **S:** You put macaroni in your chili?
65. **G:** Uh huh.

A Different Clinical Approach to Conversation

Our usual approach to conversational analysis is to look at the conversation turn-by-turn, discussing variables such as topic maintenance and turn relationships. The overall impression of many language impaired children does not suggest that a failure to abide by rules of turn taking or an inability to talk on topic is necessarily at the heart of their conversational problems. In many instances, children who have conversational problems are described by teachers or parents as "bizarre" or "confused," and it is often the case that other children avoid interacting wiith them because of their strangeness as conversational partners. What we need clinically is a way to describe this strangeness, and it does not appear that the model most often used to analyze normal adult conversations is completely useful. For this reason, we have turned to a model developed specifically for analyzing conversations of children with language impairments.

Bishop and Adams (1989), working out of a perspective developed by Rapin (1987), suggest that there may be a sub-group of language impaired children, called "semantic-pragmatic disordered," who can be identified based on their use of language in conversation. As Bishop and Adams describe these children, they are those who "may have good mastery of the formal aspects of language, but conversation does not flow smoothly, because they express themselves in an odd way, come out with unexpected utterances and seem unaware of the needs of the conversational partner" (p. 242). Their research was primarily directed toward finding out whether raters could reliably identify those features in a child's conversation that led to judgements that it was inappropriate. They identified a wide range of semantic, syntactic, and pragmatic features which led to what they call a sense of inappropriateness. In their summary of their results, they report that "children with semantic-pragmatic disorder resembled younger normal children in that they frequently misunderstood the literal or implicit meaning of adult utterances and they violated normal rules of exchange structure. In other respects however, the semantic-pragmatic group did not resemble normally developing children of any age. In particular, they tended to provide the listener with too much or too little information" (p. 241).

The conversational analysis system developed by Bishop and Adams (1989), together with another quite similar one developed independently by Damico (1991) focuses on what is inappropriate in children's conversations. In other words, these systems do not represent attempts to hold up the model of a normal conversation and ask which parts of it language impaired children cannot do. Instead, the conversation of a child with language impairment is examined in and of itself, and the question is, what is it about this conversation that causes a listener (or reader) to find it bizarre or confusing? These researchers concluded that what was needed to talk about unsuccessful conversations was an analysis scheme focused on function rather than on discrete formal elements. Their approach adheres to the first rule of good observation: Do not focus on what the child cannot or does not do. Focus instead on what the child is doing. What they give us is a system designed to facilitate clinical observation of children's unsuccessful conversations, with an eye toward phrasing goals for clinical intervention to help make conversation more successful.

What is presented here is our adaptation of the analysis system presented by Bishop and Adams (1989). It reflects the categories they found most reliable when using the system to code conversational inappropriateness in three groups of children over a nine month period. They found that language impaired 8–12 year olds had levels of conversational inappropriateness similar to levels found in language normal 4 and 5 year olds. However, the patterns of inapproprate behavior in language impaired children, particularly semantic-pragmatic disordered children, were quite different. The categorization scale presented next reflects those categories which distinguished children with semantic-

Table 3-1. Coding Categories for Analyzing Conversation

I. Expressive semantics or syntax

II. Too much or too little information

>   Too little information
>   A. Inappropriate presuppostion
>   B. Unestablished referent
>   C. Logical step omitted
>
>   Too much information
>   D. Unnecessary assertion/denial
>   E. Excessive elaboration
>   F. Unnecessary reiteration
>   G. Ellipsis not used

III. Unusual content

>   A. Topic drift
>   B. Unmarked topic shift
>   C. Sterotyped "learned" language
>   D. Unappropirate questioning
>   E. Socially inappropriate remarks

pragmatic disorder from other language impaired children as well as from younger normal children. Table 3-1 presents a summary of the coding categories.

THE CODING SYSTEM

I. Expressive Semantics or Syntax

This category refers to those utterances in which the sense of inappropriateness results from unusual syntax or semantics. As Bishop and Adams define it, "in many cases, the child appeared to have selected a wrong lexical item of the correct form class, closely related to, but not precisely corresponding to, the meaning he or she wished to convey...Semantic overextensions of this kind were observed for a range of parts of speech, especially function words (connectives, auxiliaries and prepositions)" (p. 245). Also included in this category are the overly sophisticated discourse devices (such as "well," "actually," "by the way") which some language impaired children use in inappropriate contexts. Misuse of these forms may make the child's language sound stereotypical or 'formulaic.' Finally, this category is also used to code what Bishop and Adams call "aberrant syntactic formulations," which involve difficulties putting words in the right places in sentences. The examples given below will help to clarify this category:

> **Adult:** When did you go to MacDonald's?
> **Child:** We went **because** we wanted to get hamburgers.
> [child uses **because** instead of **when**]
>
> **A:** Your mom let you play outside in the rain?
> **C:** Yes, but **before we got wet** we had to get dry again.
> [child apparently means **when we got wet**]
>
> **A:** Where will you go when you get to California?
> **C:** Well, **actually**, we're going to Disneyland.
> **A:** Have you been there before?
> **C:** **Actually**, when I was littler.
> [**Actually** appears to be a filler word of some sort, which makes this child's conversation sound strangely adult-like in some contexts and weirdly inappropriate in others.]
>
> **C:** I **always** get a shot at the doctor, but I don't get a shot **sometimes**.
> **A:** You mean you sometimes get a shot but you don't always have to get one?
> **C:** Yeah, not always.

II. Giving Too Much or Too Little Information

Seven types of problems were identified by Bishop and Adams (1989) as exemplars of this category. Our sense of inappropriateness resulting from the wrong amount of information probably comes from our belief, as phrased by Grice (1975) that good conversationalists tell the listener just what he or she needs to kow, without leaving out critical information or giving unnecessary detail. Children with semantic-pragmatic disorders seem to violate this maxim in both directions. That is, sometimes they tell the listener so little that confusion results, and sometimes they go into far more detail than a question or context warrants. The following subcategories are coded:

A. Inappropriate presupposition

This occurs when the child apparently assumes that the listener has information that makes ellipsis appropriate, when in fact, such information is lacking. An example can be seen in the conversation with George:

> **A:** Do you cook chili too?
> **G:** Uh huh. Macaroni.
> **A:** You put macaroni in your chili?
> **G:** Uh huh.

In the exchange about chili, George's response of "macaroni" would have been appropriate had the adult asked "What do you put in your chili?" In the absence of such a question, however, his remark was an inappropriate use of ellipsis.

B. Unestablished referent

This is coded when a child introduces a term whose reference has not been sufficiently well established for the listener to understand the meaning. These terms are usually, but not always, pronouns. Again, the conversation with George provides examples:

> **G:** I ask the family ... what they're going to have ... bacon.
> **A:** What family?
> **G:** Marianne next door.
> **A:** Oh, you asked the family next door what they were going to have?
> **G:** You ever met her?
> **A:** No, I don't know Marianne. She's your neighbor?
> **G:** Uh huh.

This exchange is surely one of the most confusing in the entire conversation with George, partly because his initiating remark represents an unmarked topic shift, and also because the phrase the family implies a shared reference which does not exist. Further examples of George's use of unestablished reference can be seen in the pronoun use in his description of how to cook eggs:

> **G:** Put butter ... then put **those** away, melts, dip an egg and crack it. Put **it** in wastebasket. Put **it** up and push it up a little bit like the rest of the eggs.

C. Logical step omitted

This occurs when a child leaves out a logical step in an argument or a critical step in a sequence. Bishop and Adams (1989) give perhaps the clearest example of this difficulty we have ever encountered:

A: What will happen if he doesn't get better?
C: He—get some medicine—and make—and make—my brother was feeling sick on Monday.
A: Right.
C: And I took my trouser off.
A: Uh huh. Why did you take your trousers off?
C: He was sick on my trouser. (p. 252)

Another example of this sort of difficulty can be seen in the conversation with George.

G: If you get right close to you the bacon will . . . pop on you.
A: Then what would happen?
G: You'll put cold water.
A: Uh huh. It'll burn you?
G: Uh huh.
A: And then you put cold water on the burn, right?
G: Right.

The extent of clarifying dialogue following George's utterance about cold water indicates the amount of information he left out: bacon will pop on you, it will burn you, and then you put cold water on the burn.

While the categories given above are coded when the child gives too little information, four other categories may be coded when too much information is given:

D. Unnecessary assertion/denial

This occurs when the child asserts or denies a fact when the listener would not normally have needed the assertion or denial. For example:

A: Will you have milk to drink with your cake?
C: And it won't spill.

A: What else will you have at MacDonald's?
C: You don't have to have french fries if you don't want to.

E. Excessive elaboration

This can occur when a child gives much more information in response to a question than is needed, or when a child gives an elaborately specific answer when a generalization would have been expected. For example, again from the conversation with George:

A: Is she gonna have bacon for breakfast?
G: Uh huh. Put eggs in it and dip in it.
A: Uh huh.

G: Then . . . twist it a little bit with a fork. If you get right close to you the bacon will, might, will pop on you.
A: (asking George about his favorite TV show) Can you tell me what happens on that program?
G: Yeah, you spill some ink. [evidently referring to a specific episode he had watched rather than giving some general statement about the show].

F. Unnecessary elaboration

This category applies to utterances in which the child repeats information already established. This is a characteristic ploy of some children, as can be seen in the following example:

A: What happens if you miss the school bus?
C: You hafta walk or call your mom.
A: Uh huh.
C: You call your mom, and she tells you you hafta walk.

G. Ellipsis not used

This category is used to code those utterances which some have characterized as "therapized," that is, those which seem to result from someone teaching a child to "use a whole sentence." Example:

A: Do you know what this is?
C: This is a red truck.

All of these violations of our expectations about the appropriate amount of information to give in a conversational turn will disrupt a conversation. Sometimes, as when too little information is given, the conversational partner is forced to do an unusual amount of questioning for clarification and scaffolding. At other times, as when too much information is given, the impression is one of strangeness and incompetence.

III. Unusual Content

Bishop and Adams (1989) describe this category as follows: "The difference between this category and other types of semantic and pragmatic problems is that the utterances coded here gave the impression that there was something abnormal about the message the child was trying to convey—not just with the way it was conveyed. Indeed the child's expression may be very clear, but the utterance seems an inappropriate or even bizarre thing to say in this context" (p. 253). Five sub-categories have been identified:

A. Topic drift

This occurs when a child seems to go off on a tangent, to talk about something that is related in some way to the topic of conversation, but not central to the focus. It can also occur when a child perseverates on a topic, refusing to shift away from it in spite of repeated efforts by the conversational partner. Two examples from George's conversation will clarify this:

> **G:** ... That's how you cook eggs.
> **A:** Yeah, that's how you cook them. Do you like robots, George?
> **G:** Yeah. I love chili.

This example shows George's unwillingness to shift away from the topic of food, in spite of a clear attempt by the adult to move on to something else. A tangential drift can be seen in the example below:

> **A:** Do you ever cook anything else? What else do you cook?
> **G:** Eggs.
> **A:** Uh huh.
> **G:** I used to cry for eggs when I was little.

George's comment about crying for eggs when he was little is, in some way, related to the immediately preceding topic of cooking (he had just finished talking about cooking bacon), but it seems to come out of nowhere in the context.

B. Unmarked topic shift

This category is self-evident. Shifting topic without any conventional marking will almost always result in conversational breakdown. One very clear example from George's conversation should suffice:

> **A:** Let's see what I've got in here (takes out a small robot). This is a transformer, Goerge (twists the robot's head). Look what that did.
> **G:** I ask the family. . .what, what they're going to have . . . bacon.
> **A:** What family?

The conventional marking of topic initiation, as well as the classification of initiating bids is important to keep in mind when planning intervention for children who make moves as inappropriate as the one made by George above. These issues are discussed in Chapter 4, in the context of setting intervention goals for George.

C. Stereotyped "learned" language

Again, a self-evident category, which applies whenever a child's utterances sound fixed or memorized. Another example from George's conversation serves to show this: George and the clinician have been discussing TV shows, when he notices the person operating the camera, and says:

G: What's your name?
A: Kim
G: Kim, hi.
A: Hi, George.
G: Uh, nice to meet you.

George's stereotypical greeting routine sounds particularly strange in this context, given that Kim is an adult whom he has never met, and is not a participant in the conversation.

D. Inappropriate questioning

This is coded whenever a child asks a question which is not typical for the topic, or to which the adult could not possibly know the answer, or to which the child already knows the answer. One example from George's conversation occurs after he has introduced to topic of the family next door:

A: What family?
G: Marianne next door.
A: Oh, you asked the family next door what they were going to have?
G: You ever met her?

This question is inappropriate in the context, given that George had no reason at all to expect that the clinician should have met his next door neighbor. Bishop & Adams (1989) suggest that some children ask questions to avoid being questioned themselves, as they have learned that asking questions is a way to force the other person to take a turn. When questions are used in this way, it is almost unavoidable that they will be inappropriate, as the following example shows:

A: Can you tell me any more about the story we just read?
C: There was a bear.

A: Right. The bear was lost, wasn't he. What else do you remember?

C: Did you like that story?

E. Socially inappropriate remarks

These occur when a child makes remarks which are over-friendly or over-personal (Bishop & Adams, 1989, p. 255). Although it might be difficult sometimes to judge whether a child's remarks are inappropriate, one example can be seen in George's conversation, in the segment quoted above when he opens his conversation with Kim by saying "What's your name?" This is not a question that a child George's age would normally address to an adult he has just noticed in the room. Bishop and Adams remind us that "What may seem like loveable naivety in a primary school child starts to look like social incompetence in an adolescent, and children who regularly contravene social expectations in this way will attract negative reactions from other people, and may be regarded as naughty, rude, stupid, or mad" (p, 256).

PUTTING THE PICTURE BACK TOGETHER

How can we put all this back together to get a picture of George as a conversationalist? Perhaps most obviously we can see that George does have some conversational abilities. He can engage in smooth turn-taking. He can maintain a topic, although his contributions are likely to be minimal. He can also initiate a topic, although he does so with no conventional cues and with a bid which gives his listener little to go on with. His overwhelming lack of ability is most obvious in the area of meaning. His abilities to establish reference appear to collapse in the face of a need for elaborated meaning, and he depends heavily on adult scaffolding to make his meanings clear. His only attempts at elaboration in this conversation were heavily dependent on event scripts, and frequently marked by inadequate presuppositions. George seemed to have great difficulty with the framework of talking about what happened on his favorite TV shows. It is tempting to say that he wasn't interested in the topic, but this ignores the issue of his frequently inappropriate moves within this framework, such as appearing to give an isolated event from a specific episode when asked to "tell me what happens on that show." His inappropriate move suggests that he is unaware of the conventions of this framework. When he moved, in turn 30, to shift the frame, apparently to some sort of event recounting, his inability to create shared reference became particularly evident. Event recounting is perhaps the earliest of all the uses of elaborated language, and most four year olds with normal language development are able to do it with little adult scaffolding. George does not appear to be able to transfer his event knowledge to the conversation in order to use it as a basis for negotiated meaning. These are the conclusions we will attend to as we develop intervention plans for conversational problems in Chapter 4.

SUMMARY: ASSESSING CHILDREN'S CONVERSATIONAL ABILITIES

1. Obtaining a Conversational Sample

With whom should the child talk? This depends in large part on what sort of sample you want. Certainly, the conversational partner should be familiar to the child, and a person with whom the child feels at ease. Adult/child conversations are likely to be more structured, but the disadvantage is that the adult may have more difficulty not scaffolding for the child, and if you want to observe conversational breakdowns, this scaffolding will get in the way. Child/child conversations, on the other hand, may be more natural, but if you want to observe specific frameworks or topics, it will be more difficult for children to manipulate these. Generally speaking, we opt for conversations with familiar adults when we are attempting to get a sample to analyze. We will warn the adult in advance if we want particular topics covered or particular sorts of behavior to emerge.

What should the child talk about? To get the best conversation a child is capable of, it is usually best to allow the child to choose the topic. Most children will talk longer, and more freely, about topics they themselves initiate. To get the conversation started, however, the partner might want to try initiating a topic about which the child is certain to be interested. This will mean that some detective work should be done in advance, to find out what the child might want to talk about. Generic topics like TV or sports may not work with certain children, and it is a mistake to assume that all children will talk about them. Recent exciting events at home or school, unusual happenings, or strange objects which do interesting things might serve to get conversation started. Older children may be led into conversation with shared anecdotes about "the scariest thing that ever happened to me" or "the time I thought I was going to die." The rule of thumb here is to maximize the child's participation by building on his interests and his world knowledge.

What frameworks should be examined? Again, this depends on what you're trying to find out. The best way to examine a child's framework participation is to observe the child in the naturally occurring frameworks on the playground and in the classroom. In gathering a formal conversation sample, you might want to examine event recounting, problem solving, or using language to get information. Generally, we try to get at least two frameworks into every conversation sample, just to see what happens when the framework shifts.

2. Analyzing the Sample

Start with the macrostructure, and move to more detailed analysis. First, code the frameworks, and note on the transcript when these shift, and who attempts the shift. Second, code the topics, and note on the transcript when these shift, and who initiates the shift. Note whether the partner follows the topic shift. Then go through the transcript and mark any turn in which the child's behavior is inappropriate or bizarre. Trust your instincts here—if it strikes you as strange, it's probably strange. It is a good idea to have a videotape of the conversation at this point, because prosody and nonverbal behaviors such as eye contact and gesture may contribute to your assessment. Once you have noted points where the child's behavior seems inappropriate, go back to the variables listed in Table 6-1 and code the inappropriate behaviors. Then, just as we did with George, you can attempt to put the analysis together to make a summary. Does the child have difficulty with particular frameworks? Can the child follow framework shifts, or does his conversational behavior become inappropriate at these points? Can the child initiate topics? [See Chapter 4 for some additional information about coding topic initiations.] Can the child follow the topic shift when others initiate topics? Does the child make proper presuppositions? If not, is there too much information, or too little? Can the child negotiate meaning in the conversation, or do you find frequent use of inadequate reference? All of these questions should be answered as you prepare to plan intervention goals and activities.

C H A P T E R   4

Intervention with
Conversation Problems

In this chapter, we will present our ideas about how to work with children who are having problems with conversation. First, though, there are some general caveats that apply:

1. There are a variety of reasons why children might have problems with conversation. What works for one child might not work for another, so it pays to be flexible.
2. Conversational problems can appear in children at any age. Younger preschool children may not be perceived as having problems in this area because we expect less of them as conversationalists. Conversely, adolescents may be perceived as having quite severe problems, although their behavior may be much the same as that seen in 7 or 8 year olds. Our expectations for what children should be able to do shift as the children get older.
3. Talking with children about conversation may seem awkward, because we are at one and the same time "doing" conversation and conversing about it. This is the essence of metalinguistic processing, and it may not be easy for some children (or for some clinicians) at first.
4. Working with a child on conversational skills will demand that the SLP serve as a coach and a mediator rather than as a conversational partner. The natural tendency of adults when acting as conversational partners is to scaffold and compensate for the child's conversational deficiencies. This natural tendency must be resisted in order to help the child identify the points where conversational problems appear. Involvement of a third party to serve as a partner and use of videotape will be helpful.

INTERVENTION APPROACHES

When we begin to determine goals and plan remediation in the area of conversation, it is important that we choose goals and techniques that will maximally enhance the child's communication. The target behavior chosen for intervention should reflect some rule which can be generalized across contexts and situations. As we can see from the conversational sample taken from George in Chapter 3, a child who has problems with conversation is not likely to have just one problem. The aspects of conversation we have discussed are combined in interaction, and the clinician must determine which aspects are most important for each individual child. In some cases, this will mean working on some aspect designed to reduce the child's level of inappropriate behavior. In other cases, it may mean working on some aspect designed to help the child accomplish some personally important goal, such as being able to participate in a group problem solving discussion in the classroom. The ultimate goal, of course, is to improve the child's ability to plan and execute a conversation with another person. Another way to state the goal is to say that the child will conduct a conversation without being judged "weird" or inappropriate. The long-term goal, then, is not to teach turn-taking or establishing a referent. These are simply steps on the way to the real goal.

The general techniques used in conversation intervention are: **rule teaching, observation, scripting, and role playing.** Most children of school age have enough metalinguistic ability to profit from overt teaching of rules, where these can be identified. An important part of any intervention is **mediation**, or explaining to the child exactly what you are working on and why. Part of the process of mediating is explaining any rules that apply to the aspect of language you have focused on. In some cases, it will not be possible to discover rules, because the behavior is simply too context dependent to generalize about. However, when rules can be identified, they should be made overtly clear to the child. One clinician's mediation for a session on eye contact was as follows:

Today, Chris, we're going to work on eye contact. That means where you should look when you talk to people. If you don't look at the person you're talking to every once in a while, it looks like you aren't paying attention, and that makes people upset. We'll watch a couple of videos, and talk about how the people in the videos use their eyes when they talk, and then we'll do some practicing. The rule we'll work on first is this one (puts a card on the table with the rule written on it): TO BEGIN A CONVERSATION, FIRST LOOK AT THE PERSON YOU WANT TO TALK WITH.

After making the rule clear, if this is appropriate, it is time to do some observation. Carefully selected or even specially constructed videotapes are very useful here. They are better than live observation, because you can stop the tape to focus on a single frame, or to ask a child to predict what a person might say or do next. If video is impossible in your situation, then live observation is certainly better than no observation at all. The clinician above, working on eye contact, might walk around the playground with the child at recess, helping him to focus on when people make eye contact. The observation step is one we often skip, even though we realize that not all children are risk takers. Many children prefer not to try new behaviors until they feel comfortable with them, and a big part of feeling comfortable comes from watching carefully what other people do. Structured observation gives us a chance to help the child focus on the relevant part of a situation, to help him learn the right piece of the behavior.

We have thought long and hard about ways to help children figure out what to say in certain conversational contexts, and the technique we prefer involves scripting and role playing. The disadvantages of this technique are clear, of course. The child may memorize a scripted routine, and then discover that in a real life interaction the other person doesn't stick with the script. It is true that scripts are not the best way to build in flexibility. However, we have not been able to devise a better way to give a child practice, so we persist. It is best if the scripted practice can give way rapidly to more realistic practice situations, in contexts in which the clinician can intervene to scaffold and coach, of course. One clinician's scripted role playing to help a child with conversational openings was as follows:

Script 1
Child: *Hey, you know what? I got a new Nintendo game this weekend.*
Clinician: *Oh yeah? Which one did you get?*
Child: *Tells name of game and something about it.*

Script 2
Child: *Hey, guess what? I got a new Nintendo game this weekend.*
Clinician: *Where did you get it?*
Child: *My grandma gave it to me for my birthday, and it has some great new stuff in it.*
Clinician: *Like what?*
Child: *Tells something about the game.*

The target child practiced with the clinician, as well as with a confederate brought in by the clinician, until he felt comfortable with both scripts. He then went into the classroom, and at the first opportunity, tried his opening line with another child. The response was, "Big deal, so did I." Since the child had been primed to respond to a question, he was unsure about what to say, and he just stood there. The clinician, standing by, intervened and suggested that he ask a question himself. This allowed him to continue the interaction for a few more turns, and also allowed the clinician to see that she needed to include some additional options in her script. Subsequently, the target child tried his opening with other, more cooperative children, and was able to experience some success with it, which provided the clinician with a situation for generalizing a new rule: ONE WAY TO BEGIN A CONVERSATION IS TO GIVE THE OTHER PERSON SOME NEW INFORMATION.

Whatever techniques the clinician chooses to adopt in meeting a goal for an individual child, the role of the clinician in the intervention interaction will be critical. The clinician must provide support and scaffolding, while serving as a coach to help the child recognize breakdown points in a conversation. The clinician must also collaborate with the classroom teacher and the family to assure that the child receives scaffolding in as many situations as necessary. As the child gains facility in the skills being taught, the clinician must then gradually remove the scaffolding and see that other people in the child's environment do likewise.

We will illustrate the principles we have discussed above by describing the goals that were set and the intervention activities that were planned for George, the child described in Chapter 3. His clinician was Marilyn, the speech-language pathologist you met in Chapter 2.

SETTING GOALS FOR GEORGE: REFERENCE MAKING

Before turning to a discussion of how Marilyn decided to intervene with George's conversational skills, we must add some additional information about his underlying language abilities. As we noted in Chapter 3, George's sentence structures became fragmented when he attempted to engage in a lengthy conversational turn.

Marilyn was not sure whether this resulted from an underlying problem with syntax, or whether some sort of processing difficulty was involved. She decided to use a standardized test, not to tell her whether George was language impaired, but rather to give her a conservative estimate of George's ability to use his syntactic knowledge. Testing, using the CELF-R, showed that George's receptive language score was above average for his age, and his expressive language score was only slightly below the mean, with formulated sentences (in which the child is asked to make up a sentence using a target word) being most difficult for George. Marilyn concluded from the results of this testing that George's problems with sentence structure in the conversation probably resulted from the demands associated with constructing connected utterances on a given topic in the conversational setting. She decided to try to keep the intervention setting one in which George could talk about topics he knew well, to reduce the demands of the task as much as possible.

Marilyn's first step in setting goals for George was to give some thought to his ability to manipulate meaning within a conversation. She noted that it was impossible to tell whether he was even aware of making presuppositions, because his problems with establishing reference were so overwhelming. As for negotiating meanings, she saw some possibilities as long as George was able to talk within the confines of known event scripts. Framework appropriateness was an area in which she felt sure work would have to be done, given George's stereotypical attempts to enter into conversations with other people, and his inability to participate in group problem solving sessions in the classroom. These behaviors suggested to her that George was either unaware of the demands of these frameworks, or else unable to meet these demands during an ongoing conversation. Marilyn also talked with his teacher and with his mother about what aspect of his conversational behavior they believed contributed most to his conversational breakdown. They all agreed that his difficulty establishing reference was particularly striking, resulting in the need for frequent clarification and elaboration by his conversational partner.

Training conversational referential skills is by no means a straightforward or simple operation. Generally speaking, we know that by first grade, children are capable of providing adequate, unambiguous messages to listeners, particularly when they can use contextual support and have listener feedback to help them. However, they are not very good listeners at this age, in the sense that they have great difficulty deciding whether a message they receive is ambiguous. This appears to be a function of the child's monitoring abilities. Research (Robinson & Robinson, 1976) suggests that when communication fails, children routinely attribute this failure to the listener. They seem not to realize that the message may have been ambiguous or inadequate. The ability to monitor a message and determine whether it is adequate develops along with the child's metalinguistic awareness (Robinson & Whittaker, 1987). (Factors which affect metalinguistic awareness are discussed in Chapter 7).

Lloyd, Camaioni, and Ercolani (in press) conducted a study of referential communication by 6-and 9-year-old English and Italian children, and concluded that "all children performed better as speakers than as listeners and that older children were significantly better than younger children in both roles" (Lloyd, 1994, p. 63). Bryan, Donahue, and Pearl (1981) found that throughout the elementary school years, learning disabled children were behind their normal peers in the ability to compose unambiguous descriptions, repair communication breakdown, and ask for needed information when a speaker's message was inadequate. Bishop and Adams (1991) found that the performance of language impaired children between the ages of 4 and 12 years old on referential communication tasks was also behind that of their normal peers.

In setting up an intervention program for this problem, Marilyn first asked herself what she hoped to achieve with George. She realized that simply teaching him to perform adequately on a referential communication task would not necessarily carry over into real conversational situations. However, she also believed that if she could focus his attention on reference making as a reason why conversational breakdowns occurred, and provide feedback for him immediately, in a conversational setting, she might help him to develop his own self-monitoring skills. She decided, however, that George first needed to be focused in on how to make and how to detect the appropriate distinctions in less complex situations than conversations. With this in mind, she stated the long-term goal:

> **Goal:** George will increase his conversational skills by improving his ability to establish his referent, providing appropriate background information for the listener.

She then identified the interim objectives associated with this goal, based on the work of Sonnenschein and Whitehurst (1984). These researchers, working with normally developing kindergarten children, found that the ability to evaluate referential adequacy in the communication of others will transfer to speaking, listening, and self-evaluation. In the words of Sonnenschein and Whitehurst, "teaching children how to speak and listen and to evaluate their own performance does not teach them what is wrong when others speak or listen poorly, whereas teaching children what is wrong in the performance of others does teach them how to speak and listen themselves" (p. 1943). This finding led to the sequencing of interim objectives:

1. George will correctly evaluate the communication behavior of speaker and listener in a referential communication task presented on videotape.

2. George will provide sufficient information to enable a listener to distinguish among possible referents in a referential communication task in which he is the speaker.
3. George will ask for further information in the face of ambiguous messages when he functions as the listener in a referential communication task.
4. George will use his referential communication skills in spontaneous conversation with his peers.

Teaching Referential Communication Skills

Activities designed to meet the first goal involved the use of a series of staged, videotaped interactions in which two children played a "communication game." (Note: If setting up a videotape of this sort is not possible, the roles can be played by the clinician or by a confederate in the intervention session itself. The use of videotape is preferable, because it allows the clinician to concentrate on George and his responses. The videotape can be put together using home video equipment, and might make a nice project for older children in the school, if desired.) The game was explained to George as follows:

> *These two children are looking at some pictures.* [Several pages of pictures, which were shown on the videotape, were of arrays of stars of different colors and sizes.] *Fred is going to point to one of the pictures, and tell Mary something about it. Mary will have to decide whether she can pick out the right picture, or whether Fred needs to tell her more about it.*"

The first example of interaction between the children involved effective communication. For example, the children were looking at an array of stars, which differed only in terms of color, with one star of each color. While Mary hid her eyes, Fred pointed to a red star, and said, "I'm pointing to the red star." George was then asked, "Can Mary point to the same star as Fred?" Whether George was correct or incorrect, the rule for describing differences between a referent and its context was explained to him.

RULE: THE SPEAKER MUST TELL THE LISTENER WHAT MAKES THE TARGET OBJECT DIFFERENT FROM ALL THE OTHERS.

Marilyn made sure, with each set of pictures, that George was able to perceive how the objects might be distinguished from one another, and that he could talk about these features without difficulty. Then ten more exemplars were given, contrasting effective and ineffective communication (ineffective communication, in the context given above, would involve Fred saying "I'm pointing to the star," while pointing to a red star). George was given feedback after each examplar, designed to help him understand the rule. As George improved his evaluations, the language needed to differentiate the referent became more complex. The array of pictures used contained multiple red stars, for example, which had to be differentiated in terms of location on the page or in terms of size. In this situation, Fred had to tell Mary, "I'm pointing to the red star which is at the bottom of the picture," or "I'm pointing to the smallest red star." Inadequate communication in this situation would involve utterances like, "I'm pointing to the red star," or "I'm pointing to the star." George continued to receive feedback about whether his answers were correct and why. When George had become successful at evaluating the performance of other speakers, making no more than one evaluation error in ten trials, Marilyn began to show tapes on which Mary responded. Mary either pointed to the star she thought Fred was pointing to, or said she needed more information. George was asked to evaluate Mary's performance by saying whether she should have pointed, or asked for more information. As before, feedback was given after each trial, with the explanation being that if Fred did not tell Mary enough, Mary must ask for more information. George was given a new rule:

RULE: IF YOU CAN'T TELL WHICH OBJECT THE SPEAKER IS REFERRING TO, YOU MUST ASK FOR MORE INFORMATION.

When George was able to evaluate both speaker and listener roles correctly 90% of the time, using a tape with two different children, Marilyn moved to the next objective.

In the next stage, Marilyn told George that he was going to play a communication game with another child. He was shown a photograph of a boy his age, named Jeff. Using the same arrays of objects used in the videotape task, Marilyn said to George, "You have to tell Jeff something about the red star so that when he hears the tape recording of what you said, he will be able to pick it out." On alternate trials, George was told that he would hear a tape recorded message from Jeff, after which he would have to either say "I need more information" or point to the star Jeff was describing. Feedback was given to George after every trial, and trials were ordered so that the necessary information demanded more complex linguistic expression as George proceeded through the trials. After ten speaking trials and ten listening trials with feedback, George was given a trial tape with a new array of pictures, in which he played both speaker and listener roles five times, without feedback, to evaluate his performance. Marilyn's rule was that if he did not complete the trial tape with 90% correct responses, training would resume. When George had successfully completed a trial tape, giving adequate information in the speaker role and responding appropriately in the listener role 90% of the time, Marilyn moved on to the next objective, which involved putting George into more realistic settings.

George became a member of the "conversation club." Once a week in George's classroom, the teacher gave the children half an hour of "free time," during which they could choose which activities they wanted to do, from a list given by the teacher. Some of the choices involved reading to kindergarten children (the "reading club"), helping first grade children with their rote math skills by using flash cards (the "math club"), or joining the speech-language pathologist to learn American Sign Language so they could communicate with a hearing impaired child in another classroom (the "communication club"). The conversation club was established after consultation between the speech-language pathologist and George's teacher. Its purpose was to provide George with a group of two or three peers for conversation. Students were told that they would be practicing ways to have better conversations. Marilyn served as a coach for George in these interactions, by choosing the topic and announcing it in advance for all the children, having practiced it in advance with George, paying special attention to his referential skills and helping him to evaluate how well he did. During these practice sessions, Marilyn stopped George whenever there was inadequate reference, asking him for more information. She concentrated on not helping George in the way the clinician did in the sample conversation presented in Chapter 3. Had that sample conversation been a practice session, the exchange that follows should replace turns 5–7:

> S: *Can you tell me what happens on that program?*
> G: *Yeah, you spill some ink.*
> S: *I don't have enough information to understand that, George. Can you give me some more information?*

In choosing topics for the conversation club, Marilyn knew that it was important not to place demands on George to talk about unfamiliar or difficult content. Some sample topics she chose were "What's your favorite subject in school? Why do you like that subject?" or "What did you watch on TV last night?" or "Who is the best teacher you have ever had and why do you think this person was the best?" The children were also asked to suggest topics for conversations. Conversations of the club were occasionally videotaped, and George and the speech-language pathologist used these tapes to evaluate his referential skills. It was necessary to work at this level for a considerable period of time, since George had some difficulty handling this more complex task. Marilyn also arranged that during this stage, George's teacher and his family learned to say to him, "George, I'm not sure what you're talking about. Can you give me some more information?" Since the natural inclination of an adult in conversation with a child is to "fill in the blanks," this was not easy for his teacher or his family members, and they were encouraged by getting frequent reports about how important this kind of responding was for George.

Some notes about this activity

The initial training and evaluation sessions in which George was working on referential communication did not take more than 15 or 20 minutes per session, so it was not necessary to pull George out of class for big chunks of time. Frequent short sessions are probably best when working on tasks like the reference game described above, to prevent boredom or burnout on the child's part. When actual conversation practice begins, half-hour sessions may be needed. Even then, however, it is probably a good idea to switch tasks from time to time. This means that additional goals might be established for the child, either having to do with conversation or with other aspects of his language, depending on what he needs. These goals might be met in the classroom, or on the playground. One example of playground based intervention is given below.

AN ACTIVITY FOR THE PLAYGROUND

George's mother and his teacher both noticed that he had trouble initiating interactions with other children. When his routine of "Hi, what's your name" was over, he had no idea what to do next. Marilyn decided to design an intervention activity directed toward the following long-term goal:

George will improve his conversational skills in social situations to enable him to initiate and maintain an interaction in a play setting.

The interim goals involved increasing the amount of time George could sustain the interaction, from one minute to three minutes, to an unspecified period based on the natural termination of the play activity.

Marilyn began this section of the planning by observing George on the playground and in the classroom. His strategies for initiating interaction varied. At times, he would walk up to a group of children and simply stand silently watching and listening. At other times, he would approach an individual child, and invariably begin by saying "Hi." When the other child responded "Hi," George's next move would be "What's your name?" When the child responded with a name, George would answer, "Hi, Jeff [or whatever name he had been given]." And that was that. If the other child happened to be skilled enough to ask George his name, he would respond appropriately, but the interaction would usually end at that point. It was clear that George needed some more prospective moves, designed to give the other party in the interaction something to talk about. So, Marilyn set up an observation exercise for George, using a couple of confederates who were in the speech-language pathologist's caseload but were more socially skilled than George. She followed this by some role playing. The activities she designed were as follows:

She decided to capitalize on George's tendency to stand and observe what other children did on the playground. She enlisted the help of a couple of fifth grade girls who were both language impaired but were socially adept and well liked by their peers. She explained to them that she wanted them to help with a game at recess. The game involved having them act as "playgound guides" for George. One girl accompanied George, and she had a notebook and pencil to take notes. It was agreed that George would tell the note-taker what to write down. The other girl agreed to go up to groups of her friends and start conversations with them. The speech-language pathologist walked slightly behind George and his guide, who were taking notes on what the interactor said when she approached a group. (Marilyn had originally intended to have George take notes, but she discovered that if he had to write, he forgot to observe.) The speech-language pathologist was there to help mediate in case any group of children asked questions about what was happening, and also to observe herself what strategies the children used. She also tried to see to it that the girl responsible for initiations moved around from group to group on the playground, rather than staying with the first group she encountered. This game was played at recess for two days. Then George and Marilyn met to discuss the results. George's notes were not terribly complete, but they were supplemented by Marilyn's observations. Together, they identified three opening moves George could try: (1)"What are you doing?" to be used when the activity was not immediately obvious; (2)"What's that?" to be used when the play involved an unfamiliar object (one group of children had been playing with a model spacecraft, another group had built robots which they had brought onto the playground); (3)"Who's ahead?" to be used after observing any game which involved competition, such as football, baseball, or soccer.

The next stage involved having George walk around the playground with the speech-language pathologist, observing groups of children and telling her what opening he might use if he wanted to talk with them. She provided feedback, and was pleased to see that on a couple of occasions, George actually came up with some opening lines of his own that would work. They agreed that, during the next recess, George would try one opening move with children from his class, and would then come back to tell her what happened. He chose to approach a group of girls who were drawing a complex diagram in chalk on the sidewalk, and asked them "What are you doing?" They obligingly explained a new form of hopscotch to him, and asked if he wanted to learn how to play. This was a fortunate trial interaction, in that George chose a group of children who were open to his presence and willing to act as teachers for him. Following this experience, George continued to practice, sometimes with the speech-language pathologist nearby to help him with follow-up moves to keep the interaction going. The children in George's class soon became accustomed to his practice on the playground, and several asked the teacher what was happening. This led to an invitation from the teacher to Marilyn to come into the classroom and present a 20 minute lesson on making conversation, in which she focused on making prospective moves, or, as she put it, "giving the other person something to talk about. "

TEACHING ABOUT CONVERSATION IN THE CLASSROOM

Marilyn and the teacher first discussed the conversational competence of the children in the classroom, focusing on where they seemed to have the hardest time. They agreed that, while many of the children (particularly some of the girls) were poised and accomplished conversationalists, others had trouble sustaining interactions. Marilyn pointed out that any child could sustain an interaction simply by throwing the ball back into the other person's court, and that if the children knew how to give the other participant an opening, they might have an easier time. She explained to the teacher that conversational turns could be characterized in terms of their prospectiveness, The categorization of conversational bids is based on the work of McTear (1985). He classifies conversational moves in terms of the function they serve in the ongoing discourse. Directives are requests for action, such as "Look at mine," or "I need a knife." Informatives are statements that do not require response, but often receive some indication of attention, such as

"I got green," or "Mine's all done." Elicitations are requests for a verbal response. Both questions and summonses are included in this category, e.g., "Who took my stickers?" and "You know what?" Vocatives are attention getting utterances such as "Teacher" or "Mary." Wells (1981) suggests that conversational moves can be thought of as occupying different slots on a scale of prospectiveness. At one end of the scale are soliciting moves, which demand that the other person respond. Questions are highly prospective moves. At the other end are utterances Wells classifies as acknowledgements, such as "oh" or "alright." They don't give the other person anything to go on with. In the middle are utterances such as declaratives, which do not demand responses, but do not cut them off either. Marilyn proposed that they help the students with the concept of prospectiveness. To begin the lesson, Marilyn explained to the class that she and the teacher were going to do some role-playing, and she invited them to try to decide what was wrong with what they were about to hear and see. She explained that she would be the child, and the teacher would be the mother. Then Marilyn and the teacher had the following conversation:

> **T:** *[To Marilyn]: Hi. What are you doing?*
> **M:** *Nothing much.*
> **T:** *How was school today?*
> **M:** *OK.*
> **T:** *Did you pass your math test?*
> **M:** *I don't know.*
> **T:** *Was it hard?*
> **M:** *Not too.*
> **T:** *So what else happened?*
> **M:** *Not much.*

By this point in the conversation, many of the children were smiling or laughing, and Marilyn turned to the class and said, "Do you think I really wanted to have that conversation?" The children agreed that she sounded uninterested or bored. Then she asked, "What could I have done to make it better?" Responses varied from "You could have talked more," to "You could have answered the questions." Marilyn then said:

> *The problem with what I did was this: I didn't help your teacher to keep the conversation going. Everything I said was a dead end. She had to do all the work, and I just did the bare minimum. If I really wanted to talk to her, what I needed to do was try to help her a little. I needed to make my turns "prospective." A prospective turn is one that helps the other person know what to say next. There are two good ways to be prospective. One is to ask a question, and the other is to add some new infor-*

mation about the topic. I'm going to divide you into pairs, and give you a written copy of the conversation we just had. I have divided it up so that it actually looks like the beginning of several conversations. What I want you to do is decide how to make my turns more prospective."

The children had a lively discussion, and after they had agreed on some strategies, several of them were asked to share their "revised" conversations, for the rest of the class to evaluate. During this exercise, Marilyn worked with George and his partner (another boy who was not a particularly adept conversationalist), coaching them in the task. The teacher walked around the room, answering questons and evaluating what the other children were doing. One group's response was as follows:

T : Hi. What are you doing?
M: Nothing much. [revised]: Just trying to forget about what a horrible day I had.

T: How was school today?
M: Ok. [revised]: Worse than ever. Do you think we could have a law against math and math tests?

T: Did you pass your math test?
M: I don't know. [revised]: I don't know. There were 7 problems I couldn't do.

T: Was it hard?
M: Not too. [revised]: It was the hardest test I ever took. Do you like math?

T: So what else happened?
M: Not much. [revised]: We played softball at recess and Todd got hit with a bat.

SETTING GOALS FOR GEORGE:
TOPIC INITIATION AND MAINTENANCE

Language impaired children may have several sorts of problems with conversational topic. On the one hand, very reticent children will fail to introduce topics at all, and will not be able to maintain topic over more than one or two turns. On the other hand, more talkative children, like George, will introduce topics, but will fail to indicate topic shifts during a conversation. As the analysis of George's conversation in Chapter 3 indicated, failure to mark topic shifts will almost inevitably result in conversational breakdown. When a language impaired child has problems with topic, we often conclude that the child doesn't understand conversational rules. While this may be true for some children, it is more likely that cognitive or linguistic difficulties are at the root of the child's problem. Cognitive difficulties will come into play when a child simply lacks the world knowledge needed to contribute to a particular topic, or lacks the ability to organize that knowledge. Scripts and other frameworks can be useful for helping the child to call up relevant knowledge. As Mentis (1994) points out, when working with school-aged children, we should be aware not only of the child's knowledge of those scripts that organize event representations (see Chapter 5), but also of those which organize particular types of discourse, such as stories or arguments.

Linguistic difficulties will arise when a child lacks either the vocabulary or the syntactic knowledge needed to mark topic maintenance and topic shifting appropriately. Several linguistic devices may signal topic initiation (Lund & Duchan, 1988). These include:

1. Phrases of introduction, such as "That reminds me," "Speaking of _____," "You know _____, well, _____," "by the way."
2. Determiners showing first mention of a topic, such as "this X," "that X," or "those Xs."
3. Left dislocation, as in "my dog, he catches squirrels."
4. Questions, such as "You know what?" or "Do you have any brothers or sisters?"
5. Referent specification, as in "the big boy across the street." Modifiers are used to indicate that the topic is being narrowed or focused to include the modified information.

Topic maintenance occurs if, after a topic is introduced, succeeding turns adhere to that topic either by simple repetition or by adding new information. We recognize topic maintenance not only through related content, but also through such linguistic devices as ellipsis ("Who hit you on the head? He did."); pronominalization; use of definite articles ("the boy" implies that we already know which boy is being discussed); lexical reiteration, and preverbal position (noun phrases that occur immediately before the verb tend to convey information that the listener already knows).

If a language impaired child has difficulty with topic initiation or with topic maintenance, it will be important to determine whether the necessary linguistic devices are a part of the child's repertoire, and if not, to focus on one or two of them and teach the child to use them. This may result in somewhat stilted topic management during conversation, but even the repetitive use of a single marking device is better than a failure to mark topic shifts at all. It will, of course, be critical to make sure that the child understands the function of the lexical or syntactic form being taught.

After analyzing George's conversational behavior, Marilyn decided that he had several event scripts that would help him to structure conversation on particular topics. One of them, involving cooking, can be seen in the conversation reported in Chapter 3. She found, by talking with him, that he also had a clear script for visiting the doctor's office with a sore throat, for getting lunch in the school cafeteria, and for studying for and taking a spelling test. She decided to use these scripts to help support George's topic management, with the following goal:

George will mark his topic shifts in conversation with an appropriate linguistic device.

The specific objectives she laid out were as follows:

1. George will identify the ongoing topic of a conversation between other people when asked to do so.
2. George will identify the topic of a conversation in which he is a participant when asked to do so.
3. George will identify the point in a conversation when the topic is shifted when observing conversations between other people.
4. George will identify the point in a conversation when the topic is shifted when he is a participant in the conversation.
5. George will learn to use the phrase "You know what" to introduce a new topic into a conversation.

Teaching Topic Identification

Marilyn structured her intervention using the techniques laid out earlier in this chapter: rule teaching, observation, scripting, and role playing. She began her work with George by focusing his attention on conversational topic. She had videotaped several brief conversations between pairs of children in George's classroom, and she began by asking George to watch the video with her. After they had watched it once, and George had commented on who was talking and where they were, Marilyn said to him, "OK, we're going to watch it again, and after every conversation, I'm going to stop the tape and ask you what they're talking about." She did this, and, because she had chosen brief segments in which the topic of the conversation was obvious, George was able to tell her. She then said,

Another way to ask what people are talking about is to use the word "topic." The topic of a conversation is what the people are talking about. So, if I say to you "What is the topic?" you would tell me what the people are talking about. Let's try another one.

When she was certain George could identify the topic of a conversation between other children in an observation task, she then moved on to conversations in which he was a participant. She asked several children from his class to help her, and she videotaped conversations in which the children talked individually or in groups of two or three with George about topics she introduced. She began each conversation with a question designed to set the topic, such as "How do you get home from school every day?" or "If you could be another person, who would you choose to be?" She videotaped the entire conversation around each topic, knowing she would certainly have use for the conversations later on. Then she sat down with George and played the first few turns of each conversation asking him to tell her the topic of the conversation. When George could do this task, she moved on the the next stage of intervention.

Some notes about this activity

While the activity outlined above may sound overly simple for some children, we have included it because telling the topic of a conversation is as complex as telling the main idea of a paragraph. It is an advanced sort of classification task (see Chapter 8), and for some children, especially those with cognitive involvements, it presents overwhelming problems. Like many of the tasks we use in this book, this one also demands a certain metalinguistic awareness (see Chapter 7). The child must use language to analyze language. Some children can do this as long as they themselves are not involved in the interaction, but cannot do it if their own talk is the focus of the analysis. This is the reason we have broken the analysis task into two segments. While it is true that normally developing preschool children can maintain the topic of a conversation without necessarily being able to tell what the topic is, it is not possible to teach topic maintenance to a child who isn't doing it without being able to talk about what the topic is. Language teaching inevitably puts some demands on a child that normal language learning may not involve. It is possible, however, that bringing language form and use to the forefront of the child's awareness may actually facilitate learning by the language impaired child, who has not been able to learn in the more ordinary fashion.

Teaching Topic Shifting

When George was able to talk about and identify conversational topics, Marilyn moved to the next stage in the intervention process. She explained to George:

> When we have long conversations with people, we will sometimes talk about more than one topic. Moving from one topic to another in a conversation is called topic shifting. I'm going to show you a videotape of a conversation I had with a boy from another class, and we'll see if we can tell when the topic shifts.

Marilyn showed George a videotape of a conversation she had conducted with a fifth grade boy who was a fluency client. She liked the tape because, apart from his fluency problems, this child was a good conversationalist with interesting things to say. She had previously analyzed the tape, looking for topic shifts, and had identified three topics being discussed: what is your favorite sport, shifting to what games do you play after school, shifting to what foods do you like to eat most. Each topic shift was clearly marked, being indicated by a question from her to the child. She decided not to talk about the subtleties of how each topic led into the next, but rather to focus entirely on noticing when the topic shifted. She and George watched the tape once, and then went through it again with Marilyn indicating, "the topic shifted right there, George." They then went through the tape again, and Marilyn asked George to tell her what each topic was. Marilyn then explained to George:

> When you want to shift the topic in a conversation, it is important to let the other person know. If you don't let them know that you're shifting the topic, they will be extremely confused. They will not understand what you're talking about. There are lots of ways to let people know that you want to shift topic. We're going to focus on one. You can use the phrase "You know what." That will let the other person know that you're about to talk about something else. We're going to practice some conversations, so you can learn to use that phrase.

Marilyn then introduced George to what she called "the topic game." The rules of the game were simple. They would agree that two topics would be covered in the conversation, and they would identify what the topics were to be by drawing slips of paper with topics written on them out of a box. The topics they drew would be left out on the table, to remind them. Then Marilyn would begin the conversation, and after they had each talked at least twice, George could shift to the second topic, using his topic shifting phrase. George found this game quite difficult, because he had to focus both on taking at least two turns and on shifting the topic. To lessen the monitoring load, Marilyn explained to George that she would ring a bell, and that any time after he heard the bell, he could shift the topic if he wanted to. She encouraged him not to do it right away, saying that she wanted to see whether he could take her by surprise. Marilyn found that, over time, if the initial topic was sufficiently interesting, George could continue for several turns after hearing the bell, before he shifted the topic. After several weeks of practice, George remembered to use "you know what" almost every time before he shifted topics, and Marilyn decided to begin teaching him another strategy. Because George was good at formulating questions, she focused on using a question as a topic shifting device. She explained that he could introduce his new topic by asking a question about it. Using the topic shifting game they had already learned to play, she gave him the example of shifting from the topic of eating at Mac-Donald's to skateboards. She explained that he might introduce the topic of skateboards by asking "Did you ever ride on a skateboard?" or "Do you like to ride on a skateboard?" or "Do you think it's fun to ride a skateboard?" They agreed to alternate being responsible for topic shifting, to give Marilyn a chance to do some modeling for George.

After George had mastered two strategies in the game context, Marilyn decided to move to a more realistic situation. She brought back the conversation club, which George was familiar with from previous work with her. She changed the nature of the topic shifting game as follows: Each of the four children in the game, including George, would draw a piece of paper from her hand. Three of the pieces of paper were blank, and one contained a new topic. She would begin the conversation by introducing her own topic. The children would converse with her, and the child who had drawn the paper with a new topic would be responsible for shifting to that topic during the conversation. At the end of three minutes (signalled by a timer), they would stop the conversation, and try to guess who had drawn the new topic and what it had been. Although no one had a problem guessing when George had drawn the new topic, he enjoyed the game enormously, and was able to participate reasonably well in guessing who had shifted the topic when he didn't draw the assignment. Marilyn videotaped several of these sessions, which she and George could analyze later to discover what strategies the other children were using.

Some notes about this activity

Marilyn found a way to make topic shifting especially salient for George with this activity, while not putting too many demands on his language or cognitive skills. She stayed with topics George knew a lot about, and she worked with syntactic forms he had within his repertoire. She was working with the four principles advocated by Mentis (1994) always in mind:

1. Structure the discourse in such a way that the target parameter is made both salient and functional.
2. Do not violate the principles of natural conversational discourse in the attempt to highlight the target parameter.
3. Make the form-function relation between the syntactic structure and the topic management function explicit.
4. Structure the conversation to provide opportunities for producing the form-function relation.

SUMMARY

In this chapter we have discussed the principles underlying conversation intervention: rule teaching through mediation, observation, scripting, and role playing with feedback. Using the information presented in Chapter 3 to develop conversational rules like the ones given in this chapter, and drawing on your own observations of what children do naturally, together with your creativity, you should be able to devise activities to work with children at various stages of linguistic and cognitive development. We have not discussed teaching children about frameworks, although our work with George to develop moves for entering ongoing conversations would be relevant. When preschool teachers teach children how to use language to settle disputes ("If you want a turn, you must ask, you don't grab the toy."), they are teaching frameworks. When classroom teachers teach older children the rules for brainstorming sessions, they are teaching frameworks. Framework teaching fits well within the strategies of rule teaching, observation, scripting and role playing we have developed in this chapter.

If you have any doubts about the value of working with children on conversational skills, consider the words of Walker, Schwarz, Nippold, Irvin, and Noell (1994): "children who have weak social skills and problematic peer relations early in their school careers are at risk for a host of negative developmental outcomes including low self-esteem, underachievement, school drop-out, juvenile delinquency, and vocational and relationship adjustment problems following secondary schooling" (p. 72). Improving a child's conversational abilities is a major part of improving social skills for language impaired children.

C H A P T E R 5

Narratives: From
Scripts to Stories

One of the most enduring human habits of mind is our need to give structure and meaning to the experiences of our lives. We are constantly constructing frameworks, making new information and new experience fit somehow with what has come before, and altering existing frameworks to accommodate new input. The frameworks we use to help us understand, remember, and recount experiences are called schemata. A schema "is an organized representation of a person's knowledge about some concept, action, or event, or a larger unit of knowledge" (Kintsch, 1974, p. 374). Our interest in frameworks and schemata is not from the perspective of cognitive scientists studying the mind, but rather from the perspective of communication specialists studying children's narratives. The narratives children listen to and use are structured by the frameworks or schemata existing in the mind. A narrative might be thought of as a verbal expression of cognitive schemata. In constructing a narrative, a child applies verbal labels to elements within the framework or schema. For complex stories and narratives, schema are embedded one within another.

This view of narratives as being expressions of cognitive schemata is shared by a number of researchers (Mandler & Johnson, 1977; Propp, 1958; Rumelhart, 1975, 1977; Stein, 1979; Thorndyke, 1977). In event recountings, schema are expressed as scripts, which represent typical, predictable sequences of events and serve to help children make predictions and inferences. One three-year-old demonstrated the power of scripts when she heard her mother talking with a friend about a party at which a very special cake had been served. The child listened quietly to a description of the cake, and then asked "Did they blow out all the candles?" It took her mother a few minutes to realize that, for three year olds, party and cake together always mean birthdays. The child was using her birthday party script to make inferences and predictions about other parties. For stories, the schemata are somewhat different. As Liles (1993) expresses it, "schema are expressed in stories as sets of hierarchically related story grammar components, usually referred to as "episodes," which may include setting, initiating events, internal responses, attempts, consequences, and reactions" (p. 870). It is story grammar knowledge which sets up for us the series of expectations we have about what a story is supposed to be like, and which aids us in our memory of stories we read and hear.

Heath (1986) discusses narratives from a somewhat different perspective. She comments that "Children learn how to recognize, anticipate, tell, read, and respond to narratives as part of their initial language socialization at home and in their primary communities" (p. 85). Thinking about narrative from the point of view of its place in society, Heath identifies what she calls four universal types of narrative, three which report factual scenes across stretches of time (recounts, eventcasts, and accounts), and stories, which she calls fictionalized accounts of animate beings attempting to carry out a goal. Heath says, "All these narrative forms bring to consciousness past or imagined experience and require gestalt-level processes of linking similarities and dissimilarities across space and time" (p. 88). She defines recounts as those narratives in which children verbalize past experiences in the presence of those who shared those experiences. These are the display narratives which appear to be peculiar to middle class, mainstream, school-oriented families. They are always prompted by an adult, and take the form of "tell grandma what we had for lunch today," when both the child and the mother know very well what they had for lunch, and the child is essentially being asked to use language to show what is known. The second genre identified by Heath is the eventcast, in which language is used to accompany or plan events. The radio or television sportscast is probably the purest example of this sort of narrative, but children use it as well in their pretend play. Eventcasting can be seen in the following interaction among a group of children engaged in role-playing or fantasy play:

Child A.: *Let's pretend that this guy was the strongest, and he could beat all the other guys.*
Child B: *Or your guy could be the fastest one, and he runs to give the messages to everybody else.*
Child C: *No, see, what if all these guys are the same and they get to be*

the team that defends the fortress. And they have to direct what all the rest of the army does.

These children are setting up a framework within which the pretend play will occur. The framework building is, in a sense, a metacognitive activity. They have suspended their pretend play temporarily to lay out the ground rules. Once they have agreed on the rules, the play itself will be resumed. Heath points out that "within such eventcasts, children must include subordination as well as some indication of hypothetical connectedness—from actions to results—as well as coordination" (p. 89). She also sees these eventcasts as forerunners of the metalinguistic commentaries children will encounter in school.

Heath's (1986) third narrative genre, accounts, is most closely related to the scripted narratives identified by other researchers. Heath defines accounts as "the preferred early narrative form that children produce spontaneously once their basic needs are met. Through accounts, individuals share what they have experienced" (p. 89). Accounts are initiated by children, rather than prompted by adults, and derive from children's experiences or thoughts. Heath acknowledges that children are not overtly taught how to give accounts of their experiences, and that they must extract from what they hear the notion that accounts must carry a predictable progression that allows the listener to anticipate what is coming. The listener to an account must be able to reconstruct the teller's mental sequence. In other words, the speaker must enable the listener to anticipate and thus comprehend what is coming. If accounts are, for the most part, based on scripted experience, it is likely that the underlying scripts of teller and listener will be to some extent similar, and thus will allow the listener to anticipate to some extent what the teller will talk about. When a child begins an account with "I had a sore throat and my mom took me to the doctor," a listener can immediately set up a series of expectations about what happened. While every account of a visit to the doctor will, of course, be individual and unique, all such visits share a certain framework within which the individualized experience occurs. It is this framework which is scripted in our minds, and which governs our account of the individual experience.

Finally, Heath (1986) discusses stories, which she says all societies have in one form or another. The key difference between accounts of events and stories is that "Fictional narratives embrace events, actors, and results that do not have to exist outside the creator's imagination" (p. 90). In our culture, stories are goal directed narratives. That is, they have a point. It is possible to say what a story is "about." In addition, stories are episodically organized. The episodes in a story are linked temporally or causally, and the components within an episode are logically related in a way that allows them to be comprehended as units rather than as a series of statements. Story structure, like the conventions governing accounts, is not taught to children but rather absorbed by them from their experience with stories. Even very young children, if they have heard stories often, can tell stories with some of the elements of conventional structure, as can be seen in this story written by a four-year-old (we have conventionalized the spelling and punctuation):

> *Once there were some bugs. They went into the deep dark woods and there they met a monster. They shot the monster. They went back into their hole. And they never went back into the deep dark woods again.*

This child knows how to begin a story, and how to end one. He also knows something about the language of stories. The use of "deep dark woods" and the proposition "into" would not be likely to occur in this child's spontaneous conversation. They are usages that occur often in fairy tales and folktales, and this child has clearly been read to enough to absorb these linguistic conventions as well as the structural conventions for stories.

In the rest of this chapter, we will consider scripts and stories in some detail, discussing children's development of these two sorts of narratives, and the kinds of performance typical of school-aged language impaired children. We will then present case studies, which will serve as a basis for narrative analysis and for our discussion of intervention in Chapter 6.

SCRIPTED EVENT RECOUNTING

A script might be defined as a set of expectations about routine events that is organized in a temporal-causal fashion (Fivush, 1984; Nelson, Fivush, Hudson & Lucariello, 1983). We use scripts as frameworks when we describe routine events, and they are important aids for our memories of specific instances of events (Bower, Black & Turner, 1979; Nelson, 1981, 1986). Nelson and Gruendel (1981) describe a script as "an organized body of knowledge such that a part implies the whole and the whole is more than the sum of the parts" (p. 138). To understand what is meant by the "part implying the whole," we have only to realize that a sentence like "Mary blew out all the candles, and then began opening the presents" will call to mind all the associated events of a birthday party. Schank and Abelson (1977) describe what is meant by saying that the whole is greater than the sum of its parts by pointing out that we apply our scripts for familiar events to other, similar events as a basis for predicting what might happen. When presented with a story about travelling on a train, children who have never been on a train but have travelled on airplanes will often be surprised that the train story does not contain a flight attendant.

The temporal-causal organization of scripts is also an important feature. The events in a script exist in a set order, which is constrained either by the fact that one event must follow another in time (you can't blow out birthday candles until they have been lighted) or logically (one would not attempt to cut a birthday cake unless the candles had been blown out first). Even very young children have scripts that are temporally or causally ordered. As evidence of this, consider the insistence of some quite young children that their bedtime routines be followed in the same order every night. While parents may interpret this "rigidity" as another maneuver in the battle over bedtime, the fact that children recall the events in a constant order is evidence of their temporally ordered mental representation of the event. Causal organization in a child's script can also be seen, even before the child is capable of verbalizing causal relationships. For example, one 2 year old was using toy furniture and people to act out her script for going to MacDonald's. She got the people into the restaurant, and then was asked "Now what do we do?" Her response was "Now we have to find the bathroom." Upon hearing this, her mother laughed and pointed out that the child was being toilet-trained, and that no matter where they went, they always had to locate a bathroom "just in case." This piece of the script was not temporally constrained; that is, it did not have to occur at some set point in the trip to MacDonald's. It was, however, causally constrained, although it is doubtful that the child could have explained the cause fully.

Development of Scripts

As we implied in the preceding paragraph, even very young children form scripted representations of familiar events. Although the scripts of younger children are less detailed and shorter than those of older children and adults, they are otherwise remarkably similar (Fivush & Slackman, 1986; Nelson, 1986; Slackman, Hudson & Fivush, 1986; Nelson & Gruendel, 1981). Nelson (1978) and Nelson and Gruenel (1986) studied script reports of 4-, 6-, and 8-year-old children. They reported that there were very few idiosyncratic events in the children's scripts, and that there was very high consistency across children in the acts that were mentioned. Hudson and Nelson (1983) investigated the script use of 4- and 6-year old children as they recalled short stories about a very familiar event (a birthday party) or a less familiar but highly structured event (making cookies). They found that at both ages, the children recalled more information from the birthday party story, but that they sequenced story units more accurately in the story about the more causally organized event of baking cookies. In general, the 4 year olds recalled fewer story units and were less accurate and consistent in sequencing the stories. They also discovered that the younger children's story recall was more affected by the inclusion of script events in the wrong order than was the recall of first graders. These results, along with those of others, suggests that development in scripts occurs from early childhood to later childhood, and that children use their scripts not only to structure their verbal accounts of experience but to aid their recall as well.

Ross and Berg (1990) point out that we should not ignore the possibility that both adults and children may have more idiosyncratic scripts than previous research has suggested. They found that the manner in which scripts were elicited affected the degree to which their subjects reported idiosyncratic information. For example, limiting the number of acts in a script (by telling the subject to list eight things that happen at a birthday party) will tend to cause subjects' scripts to be more alike. The impact of individual differences in scripts should not be minimized, particularly when script based stories or event recountings are being used in language assessment. Individual differences in scripts will have a strong influence on memory for new information, and also on comprehension. However, the more similarity between one's own script for an event and the story or account of someone else, the more facilitative the script framework will be. In fact, the influence of our personal scripts for events is so strong that we will tend to alter what we hear or read to conform with what we expect based on our own scripts. For example, if we read an account of a birthday party in which no mention is made of blowing out candles on the cake, and if blowing out the candles is a major ingredient of our birthday party script, it is likely that, if we are asked to retell the account we read, we will insert blowing out the candles. The same thing will happen in reverse if a story or account contains information that is not a part of our scripts; that is, we tend to omit information that does not fit our own frameworks.

When a child is able to use an existing script to facilitate comprehension or talking about a story, the results are striking. As Ross and Berg (1990) show, "In script contexts, children use more semantically complex language (e.g., speak significantly more often of past and future events, speak of many different topics in one conversation) and are better able to answer questions than in other contexts" (p. 41). Ross and Berg then go on to discuss the reasons for the facilitative effects of scripts. One possibility is that an existing script may reduce the processing demands of a language task, by allowing the child to concentrate on linguistic demands rather than content demands. The script provides an organizational framework for the content, and a support for recall. For this reason, language assessment is often built around tasks that will allow a child to take advantage of scripted information. A child may listen to a story about a birthday party and then be asked to retell it or answer questions about it. Or, a child may be asked to talk about "what you do when you go to MacDonald's." A child who has a highly idiosyncratic script for these events, or whose script may be shorter and less elaborated due to less varied experience, will be at a disadvantage in these situations. Before we assume that a child has a script for a given event, or that the child's script will match anyone else's, we should make every effort to elicit some information about the child's experiences. In a society as full of individual and cultural differences as ours, the assumption of commonality is frequently dangerous. Remember the 2 year old whose MacDonald's script included finding the bathroom!

Scripts and Language Impaired Children

There is little information in the research literature dealing specifically with script use by language impaired children. We have no reason to believe that cognitively normal children fail to develop scripts. It is possible to tell from a child's nonverbal behavior that scripts for familiar events are present. A child who knows what to do in the classroom, and who can predict what will happen next certainly has a classroom script, whether she can tell us about it or not. A child who plays soccer successfully, never violating rules and understanding when his team has scored and how to keep the other team from scoring certainly has a soccer script, even though his account of how to play soccer may be disjointed and unclear to us. The key here is not the presence or absence of scripts, but rather the ability to verbalize those scripts. Verbalizing a script, either in recounting an experience or in giving directions for how to play a game or how to get your lunch in the school cafeteria places demands on the linguistic system which will tax the language impaired child's abilities. Even with a script there to act as a framework, many language impaired children have trouble organizing and ordering such tasks. There are two possible explanations for this difficulty, and both may be operating.

First, it is possible that the language impaired child has difficulty attaching verbal labels to elements within the script, or retrieving those verbal labels that have been attached. A child may know perfectly well the steps necessary to get lunch in the school cafeteria, but may not have the words to talk about "the bin where the tableware is kept" or "the conveyer belt where you put your tray when you're done." Alternatively, the child may know the words, but, due to word finding difficulties, may not be able to retrieve them at will. In either case, the child's script will sound overly general, lacking in detail. It is also likely to be shorter than the scripted account of a child who is not having problems with the vocabulary needed for the account. A second linguistically based difficulty may arise due to the temporal and causal ordering of scripts. Relational terms and clausal constructions are difficult in the early elementary grades even for some children who are developing language normally. "Because" and "if/then" constructions are not usually fully developed until children are 8 or 9 years old, and even the familiar "and" conjunction may not signal full understanding by a child of underlying temporal or causal relations. Consider the following account by a first grade child of an event that occurred on the playground:

> *See, nobody wouldn't take turns on the swings, and Tiffany got mad and she pushed too hard and then Jennifer just fell out of her swing and she said she was going to tell and Tiffany started calling her baby, baby and all that.*

It is impossible to say, based on this account, what this child understands about the causal relations that are implied by the ordering of events in her account. Only probe questions such as "What was Jennifer going to tell the teacher?" or "Why did Tiffany call Jennifer a baby?" or "Why did Jennifer fall out of her swing?" would clarify the child's underlying script. Donohue and Bryan (1984) examined the narratives of a group of learning disabled adolescents, and reported that these children used fewer connectives, such as "so" or "also" than their peers, and that their narratives were generally less coherent. The inability to linguistically code temporal or causal connections will certainly influence the adequacy of children's scripted accounts of events, and possibly their comprehension of accounts given by others as well.

The second possible explanation for language impaired children's difficulty with scripted accounts of events is suggested by Westby (1984) and also found in the work of Torgeson and Goldman (1977). Westby suggests that although learning disabled children may be able to correctly answer questions about the cause/effect or temporal relations in narratives, they cannot make their own sustained narratives hold together for a listener. Without the aid of focused questions by a listener, they tend to go off on tangents and lose sight of the underlying theme or the main idea of the narrative. Westby proposes three possible explanations: that the child has an inefficient processing system, that planning and monitoring skills are lacking in these children, or that the child may actually have insufficient schema knowledge (p. 122). The first possibility would result in the child being slow to retrieve schemas or having difficulty maintaining or changing schemas as needed. The child's narrative would show response delays, difficulty changing tasks, and the need for repetitions and cues. A narrative such as this one, from a fifth grade boy, suggests such problems:

> **Adult:** Do you know how to cook?
> **Child:** Sure. I cook all the time when my mom's not home from work yet.
> **Adult:** What kinds of things do you make?
> **Child:** I can make bacon and eggs, and I make microwave popcorn a lot, and also pizza.
> **Adult:** Do you make pizza from scratch, or from the freezer?
> **Child:** We usually have some in the freezer.
> **Adult:** Tell me what you do with the frozen pizza.
> **Child:** Well, I just put it in the microwave and zap it.
> **Adult:** Do you have to take off the wrappings first?
> **Child:** Oh yeah, you unwrap it and put it on a plate or something.
> **Adult:** How do you know how long to cook it?
> **Child:** Well, you read on the package. Sometimes it's like 3 minutes or 5 minutes.
> **Adult:** What about bacon? Do you make that in the microwave?
> **Child:** Bacon on pizza, you mean?
> **Adult:** No. I mean if you want bacon and eggs.
> **Child:** Not with pizza.
> **Adult:** No. I mean, what if you wanted bacon and eggs instead of pizza. Would you cook them in the microwave?
> **Child:** Well, sometimes you can cook pizza in the regular oven, like my mom does.

This child demonstrates difficulty changing from the discussion of pizza to talking about cooking bacon and eggs, and the adult has to do considerable prompting to get anything like a complete account of how to cook pizza in the microwave.

The second possibility would be suggested if the child produced a series of sentences which, though adequate in themselves, were not organized in a coherent, systematic manner. Such narratives tend to result from problems with the "executive system" (Anderson, 1977). Children with this problem cannot plan an account in advance, and they cannot monitor the adequacy of what they are saying as they go along. Westby (1984) suggests that "these students are able to recognize schemas, but they cannot evoke them without assistance" (p. 122). The following account, given by a second grade language impaired child certainly suggests something of this sort:

Adult: *What do you like to do after school?*
Child: *Usually I just play basketball with my brother.*
Adult: *Are you a pretty good basketball player?*
Child: *Yeah, I can beat my brother and he's in fifth grade.*
Adult: *I've never been exactly sure about how to play basketball, myself. Could you explain to me how you play it?*
Child: *Well, you have a ball and a basket, or sometimes you have two baskets, and you have two teams. And you just shoot baskets and you have to be careful not to foul. Sometimes my brother fouls me and then I get to shoot free throws and I can always make them. That's why I win.*
Adult: *So, how do you score points in this game?*
Child: *You shoot baskets, and it's two points for a free, I mean a field goal and one point for a free throw. Sometimes I get to shoot two free throws and then I get two points.*

This child seems to be having trouble moving away from his own after-school experience to a more generalized account of how to play basketball. In addition, he doesn't seem to have any idea about how to proceed with the task of telling a relatively uninformed listener how to play a game. Compare his account with that of another second grader (not language impaired) telling how to play checkers:

Adult: *What kinds of things do you and your grandfather do together?*
Child: *Mostly we play checkers.*
Adult: *Who wins?*
Child: *Well, sometimes he wins and sometimes I win. But he's pretty tricky.*
Adult: *Do you know, I don't think I've played checkers since I was ten years old. I've probably forgotten how. Could you remind me how you play checkers?*
Child: *Well, you have two people, and one takes black checkers and one takes red. Then you put your checkers on the board, and you try to move to the other side. And you can jump the other person's checkers, and if you do you get to take them off. And if you get all the way to the other side, you get kinged, and kings can move in any direction. And the object of the game is to get all the other person's checkers off.*

While this account would not serve to help a person who had never played checkers, this child does seem to have some understanding of how to talk about the key aspects of the game, and does tell what the object of the game is. She demonstrates an overall concept of the game apart from individual instances of playing it. This overall scheme, combined with some sense of what the listener might need to know, makes her account more adequate than that of the previous child. The thing to remember here is that both children undoubtedly have scripts for playing these games. What we see in their accounts is not the absence of a script, but instead varying levels of ability to use the script to organize a verbal account. Linguistic competence and the ability to plan and monitor a sustained narrative come into play in tasks such as this.

The third group of students Westby discusses are those who, in her words, "lack representations for world knowledge. They can neither evoke appropriate schemas nor adequately recognize schemas presented to them" (p. 122). The assumption here is not that the child lacks the ability to form schemas altogether, but rather that the child lacks sufficient experience to have done so. It is not clear how much experience with a given event a child needs to form a script for that event. Normally developing children probably begin to script on the basis of a single encounter with an event. It is possible that some language/learning impaired children may require more experiences, or even some overt external help with structuring the experience, to know what the key or main elements are. It is important to rule out this explanation for any child who is having trouble recounting an event. The most obvious way to do this is to ask the child for an account of an event you are sure the child has participated in, such as what happens when you have a fire drill at school, or how to get lunch in the school cafeteria. Another way to be certain the child has formed a script is to look for evidence in the child's nonverbal behavior. If the child can go to McDonald's and get a hamburger, or can play checkers without making mistakes, then the script for the activity is present. One cue that a child might be having difficulty with scripting everyday classroom routine would be that the child found it necessary to watch and imitate other children, even for activities that occurred with great regularity, such as leaving the classroom to go to music or art class.

Summary: Assessing Scripted Event Recountings

Scripted event recountings occur frequently in children's communication. They are verbal manifestations of the event schemata children form from their experiences with the world. Even very young children can be seen to have scripts, based on their nonverbal behaviors. When language impaired children's event recountings are unclear or disorganized, we should not assume that the child does not have a script for the event (although this may be a possibility, especially if the child has not had experience with a given event). It is more likely that the child's linguistic or planning and monitoring abilities are causing difficulty. Any language assessment which involves narrating scripted activities should include a check to make sure the child has had experience with the targeted event, and ideally should include some attempt to discover the extent to which the child's script might be idiosyncratic, perhaps by questioning a parent or teacher. If there is any question about the child's experiential base, the event chosen for narration should be one that the child can demonstrate nonverbal competence with, such as playing a game or engaging in some school routine.

Westby (1984) also points out that it may not be possible to tell from traditional standardized tests of language whether a child has problems with scripted narratives. Many children who perform adequately on language tests which are focused on syntax or vocabulary knowledge will demonstrate difficulty with event recounting or story retelling. As Westby says, "The majority of present tests do not require that the child integrate information as is required by narration; or if the test has required such integration, the analysis procedures have not considered the integrated product—only the components of vocabulary, morphology, or syntax" (p. 123).

When asking children for scripted event recountings, it is important to be clear about whether the goal is to obtain a verbalization of the child's script, or to have the child use the script framework to tell about a particular event. In the first instance, the question used to get the child to talk must be carefully phrased. For example, if we want a script for a fire drill at school, we should ask "Tell me what you do when there's a fire drill at school," as opposed to "What happened when you had a fire drill at school?" or "Tell me about what you did when you had a fire drill." The latter two questions are much more directed toward getting an account of a specific fire drill the child participated in. We assume that the child's "fire drill script" would support and structure these accounts, but we might not get the full script by asking such questions. McCabe and Rollins (1994) suggest that, when working with younger or more reticent children, personal event narratives may be obtained by using what they call a "conversational map." This technique involves having the adult begin by sharing a brief personal narrative of her own, followed by a question designed to get the child to share a narrative on the same topic. For example, the adult wishing to obtain an account of a trip to the airport to meet a visiting grandmother might say "My husband went to New York last week on a plane. I had to go to the airport to meet him when he came home, and it was very crowded. First, I had trouble finding a parking place, and I had to walk a long way to get into the terminal. Then I had to look on the TV screen to find out where his plane would be coming in, and walk a long way to get to the right gate. I was pretty tired of walking by the time I found the right place. Have you ever had to meet anybody at the airport?" These researchers propose a scoring procedure based on a set of questions having to do with whether the child's narrative includes more than two past tense events, whether these events are sequenced in the way they must have logically occurred, and whether there is a "high point" or a concentration of evaluative comments and a resolution that winds up the narrative. The report that this scoring procedure has been shown to be both easy to use and quite reliable. As well as providing us with a way to talk about the adequacy of a child's event account, it also provides us with a good starting point for phrasing intervention goals, as we will demonstrate in Chapter 6.

STORIES

While scripts are schemata formed in the child's mind based on experience with the real world, story frameworks are dictated by stories themselves. The framework for stories exists within those narratives we call "stories," and children must extract the framework from stories they hear. There have been numerous attempts to describe story frameworks (Rumelhart, 1975; Thorndyke, 1977; Stein & Glenn, 1979). In general, all involve the presence of a setting, in which the characters and the time and place circumstances of the story are introduced, and a goal which is reached in a series of episodes. An episode consists of an initiating event, an attempt by the story's characters to deal with the initiating event, and a consequence of the attempt. The initiating event may be internal to a character, such as a decision to do something or a physical state such as feeling hungry, or it may be external, such as a fire or the receipt of a letter. Generally, the initiating event will be followed by a plan, formulated by the characters to deal with the event. This plan may not necessarily be stated in the story, but the actions resulting from the plan will be. These actions comprise the attempt section of the episode. The outcome of the attempt is the consequence section of the episode, and it may be an external event, such as the death of an enemy, or an internal event, such as a character recovering from an illness. At any point in the episode, we may also find internal responses of the characters, which are statements about emotional states or feelinlgs. Episodes in a story will be connected to each other either additively (and), temporally (then), or causally (because). Well-formed stories also have clear endings, which serve to bring closure to the episodes. We have taken a truncated version of the familiar story of The Three Little Pigs, and analyzed its episodic structure to illustrate the components of a story grammar:

Setting   *Once upon a time there were three little pigs who lived with their mother in a very small house.*

Initiating event	*One day the mother said, "You are too big to live with me in this small house.*
Initiating event	*"You must go out and find houses of your own."*
Plan	*The first little pig saw a man with a load of sticks.*
Plan	*He decided to buy the sticks to build a house.*
Attempt	*He worked very hard for a whole day.*
Consequence	*And he built a house of sticks and moved in.*
Initiating event	*One day the big bad wolf came along and saw the house made of sticks.*
Initiating event	*"Little pig, little pig, let me come in," he called.*
Internal response	*The little pig was very frightened.*
Attempt	*"Not by the hair of my chinny chin chin," said the first little pig.*
Attempt	*"Then I'll huff and I'll puff and I'll blow your house down," said the wolf.*
Consequence	*And he huffed, and he puffed, and he blew down the house made of sticks.*
Consequence	*And the first little pig ran to the house of the second little pig, before the wolf could eat him.*
Ending	*And the three little pigs all moved in together and lived happily ever after.*

This admittedly abbreviated version of the familiar children's story is put here only to make the bare bones of the story framework obvious. In its many variations, this story contains numerous episodes, with different consequences (sometimes the first and second little pigs get eaten) and different endings (sometimes the pigs boil the wolf in a pot of water after he comes down the chimney of the third little pig's house; sometimes they eat him, sometimes not). This basic setting-episodes-ending structure is characteristic of all stories in our culture, as is the presence of a plot. The plot of a story is the underpinning for the goal directed nature of the episodes, and might be thought of as "what the story is about."

Westby (1984) cites one of the first attempts to describe narrative episodes, by Propp (1958). Propp's analysis is intuitively appealing to many students because it is more clearly related to the content of stories than the Stein and Glenn (1979) approach described previously. Propp's idea is that the plot of a story is made up of what he called "functions." A function might be thought of as a character's act which has significance for the course of action of the story as a whole. He maintains that all stories are made up of a limited set of functions, and that while no story will have all of the functions, those that are included will always occur in the same order. Todorov (1971), as described by Westby, grouped Propp's functions into five metafunctions, two having to do with states of equilibrium, two with states of transition, and one with disequilibrium. As Westby describes it, "In narratives, an initial state of affairs (equilibrium 1) is changed in some way (transition 1) into a state of affairs that is opposite to it (disequilibrium). This state is then changed in some way (transition 2) so that we get back to a state that is analogous to the initial one (equilibrium 2)" (p. 113). In the Three Little Pigs story above, equilibrium 1 (the pigs live with their mother) is changed by the mother's directive that they find their own houses (transition 1) into disequilibrium (the pigs go out to build houses). Transition 2 (the wolf's blowing down of the first two pigs' houses, and their escape) changes that disequilibrium to equilibrium (the three pigs live together in the third little pig's house). This "function analysis" is a good way to capture the plot of a story. Not all stories will include all five functions, but every story must have at least three: equilibrium, transition, and disequilibrium. Sad stories will stop with the characters in disequilibrium, while happy ones will include a transition back to equilibrium again.

Development of Stories

Much of our information about children's development of story schema comes from the work of Applebee (1978). Applebee's model is based on Vygotsky's (1962) model of cognitive development, and was developed by analyzing the stories told by preschool children. Since, as Westby & Martinez (1981) point out, many learning disabled children, even in middle school, do not have the narrative abilities of 4 and 5 year olds, it will be important for us to understand how children's stories change during their early years. The basic changes may be summarized as follows:

1. Children's earliest attempts to tell stories lack both centers and relations among the events. They are basically made up of unconnected elements. Applebee calls them "heaps." The story below, from a three-year-old girl, is an example:

   A girl named Mandy went to the store. Mom said popsicles for lunch. And all the children have naps and they have hamburgers and french fries.

2. Following this is the stage Applebee calls "sequences." These are not much more advanced than heaps, but they do tend to have a central character, setting, or topic. The elements of the story will be related to this central piece through very concrete associations. The children's book *Harold and the Purple Crayon* by Crockett Johnson is an

example of a sequence story, since it consists only of Harold and the pictures he drew with his purple crayon. There are no cause-effect sequences or logical connections from picture to picture. Other sequence based stories for children are *The Snowy Day* by Jack Keats and *Gilberto and the Wind* by Marie Hall Ets. The story below, from another three-old, is also an example of a sequence:

A monster came and ate up all the people. And it ate up all the cars, and then it ate up the houses and the trees and all the people's clothes. And the boy killed it with a bomb.

3. The next level is called "primitive narratives." These stories, like sequences, have a central character or setting or topic, but in addition the individual elements are related to the central element in some complementary way. The story elements follow logically from the characteristics of the center. Westby (1984) says that primitive narratives represent the first use of inferences in children's stories, in which they go beyond concrete or obvious information and become aware of "the reciprocal causality between thoughts and events" (p.116). Such children's books as *Alexander and the Terrible, Horrible, No Good, Very Bad Day* by Judith Viorst or *There's a Nightmare in My Closet* by Mercer Meyer are examples of primitive narratives. The story below, from a four-year-old boy, is a good example of a primitive narrative told by a child:

The bear was angry because he got bit by the bees. And he tore up their house and he ate all the honey. And then the angry bear got a stomach ache. The end.

4. Applebee calls the next stage "unfocused chains." In this sort of story, the individual elements are linked through logical or cause-effect relationships, but they have no relation to a center as sequences and primitive narratives do. As a consequence of the absence of a center, there is no plot, and no basis for deciding what to include in a story and what to leave out. Westby points out that pure unfocused chain stories are rare, because once children become aware of true logical relationships, they are not only tying together the events in the story but are also tying these to some central theme or character. However, she also says that some children's books, such as *Why Mosquitoes Buzz in Peoples Ears* by Leo and Diane Dillon might be perceived as unfocused chains by children (Westby, 1982).

5. Focused chain narratives are the final stage before the development of true narratives. The focused chain is characterized by a central character and a true sequence of events, but will lack a true plot. The absence of a plot results from children's still undeveloped understanding of character motivation and goals. This means that the story's ending may be either missing or unconnected with the events

set up at the beginning of the story. Television soap operas are good examples of focused chain narratives, as are any books of the "adventures of" type, such as Beverly Cleary's Ramona stories. Most of the stories told by kindergarten and elementary school children are focused chains. It is sometimes difficult to tell that such stories are not true narratives, until the child is asked to explain why events occur in the story and is unable to explain (Westby, 1982). The following story, told by a five-year-old girl, is an example:

The princess wanted to marry the prince, and the bad king said the prince had to find a magic ring. The prince went far away and a witch came and helped him. The witch threw all the monsters into the fire, and the prince stole the horses. The horse was magic, and the prince flew over the mountains. The bad king went away in the fire. And that's all.

6. Finally, around age 5 or 6 years, children become capable of true narratives. True narratives have connected events, centers, and plots. The events may be connected either causally or temporally, and the plot will result from the motivations and goals of the main characters. The ending of the story will be related to its beginning. The following story, from a six-year-old, is an example:

Once there was a little, little fish. He liked to swim in the ocean. He swam right into the mouth of a big whale, and he didn't know what to do. So he started to bump into the big fish's teeth, and the big fish got a toothache, and he opened his mouth to say "ow." The little fish swam out and got away and he never went in a big fish's mouth again.

It is only when focused chain or true narratives have developed that we can use story grammar frameworks such as those of Stein and Glenn (1979) to analyze children's stories. Westby (1984) points out, however, that internal responses and plans may often be omitted from young children's stories. In fact, Stein and Glenn suggest that first-grade children focus primarily on settings, initiating events, and consequences. At later ages, children will include details of attempts and endings. Internal responses and plans are seldom found in the stories of children under 10 years of age.

The development of narrative skills is dependent both on cognitive development and on certain linguistic abilities. Applebee's (1978) entire classification system is derived from the cognitive theory of Vygotsky (1962), and uses changes in cognitive abilities to explain changes in narrative abilities. For example, children younger than age 5 years are in a preoperational stage and are unable to deal with more than one concept at a time, or with relationships among concepts. Because true narratives are built on logical relations among events and on relations between characters' thoughts and motivations and their actions, we should not expect preoperational children to either tell or comprehend true narratives. The transition to true narratives coincides with the cognitive transition to concrete operational thought, around age 5 years. Children in this cognitive stage are able to hold and manipulate two ideas in the mind at once. They can reverse their thought processes, engage in hierarchical categorization, and perceive part-whole relationships (Westby, 1982). Since true narratives, with their complex interweaving of episodes and the necessity for logical endings that relate back to the beginnings, demand such cognitive skills, it is not surprising that true narratives are not seen in the stories of children until kindergarten or first grade. In fact, very complex narratives may be too demanding for most children to compose until the middle elementary grades, although they may enjoy listening to or reading them. With the development of formal operational thought in adolescence, children become capable of narratives that have morals, or implications beyond the story itself. In addition, stories built around similes, metaphors, and allegories are possible.

Narrative development also is related to children's linguistic abilities. Obviously, the formation of complex sentences and the use of relational terms will make possible more complicated narratives. More importantly, the ability to divorce language use from the here-and-now, in order to talk about events outside the immediate nonverbal context is important for story telling and for story comprehension. A good story carries all its meaning in the text (see the discussion of text meaning in Chapter 7 and the discussion of presupposition in Chapter 3 for discussions of this). This means that the story teller (or writer) must be able to use explicit language to convey meaning, and that the listener (or reader) must be able to make inferences, bringing knowledge of the world to bear on the text (see Chapter 7 for an extended discussion of inferencing). As Westby (1982) says, when children tell stories, their story schemas are not separate from the linguistic structures they use. However, this does not mean that stories written for children necessarily need to use the same sorts of syntactic structures children might be capable of producing. Children's comprehension of language is generally in advance of their expressive ability, and simple sentences are not always sufficient for the sort of explicit meanings stories must convey. Stories can be simple in terms of narrative structure or vocabulary, but it is not always wise or necessary to attempt to simplify syntax when telling or writing stories for children.

Summary

Children begin to tell stories almost as soon as they begin to communicate about more than their immediate needs. However, the stories of young children are not like those of older children. Children's narrative abilities develop throughout the preschool and elementary school years. Both cognitive and linguistic development affect children's ability to tell and to comprehend stories. Children's earliest stories lack logical or temporal relations between events, and do not have centers or plots. As children mature, they include more elements of story frameworks, including not only settings, but more complete episodes and developed endings. Character motivation, planning, and the relations between attitudes or plans and events are among the last elements to appear in children's stories. These changes in narratives reflect the child's movement from preoperational thought through concrete operations to formal operations, and the development of the ability to use complex relational terms and figurative language.

Language Impaired Children and Stories

The most comprehensive study of the story grammar abilities of language impaired children is that of Merritt and Liles (1987). These researchers compared the story telling, story retelling, and story comprehension abilities of 20 language impaired children between the ages of 9 and 11 years with those of a group of age matched non-impaired peers. All the children in their study had normal performance IQ scores, and none had hearing loss or any other deficits that might account for their language difficulties. Each of the 40 children in the study completed three tasks: generating a story in response to a story stem (i.e., "Once upon a time, two friends were in a deep and dark cave..."); retelling a brief, four-episode adventure story; and answering two sets of comprehension questions, one set designed to assess comprehension of factual information about characters and events and one set designed to assess the child's understanding of the relations among the events in the story. Merritt and Liles found that while all the children in their study told stories with both complete and incomplete episodes, there were some differences between the two groups. In both the story generation and the story retelling tasks, the children in the control group produced more complete episodes and a higher frequency of story grammar components than the language impaired children. During both story generation and story retelling, the language impaired children's incomplete episodes were likely to contain initiating events, but the result or consequence segment of the episode was likely to be omitted. In the story retelling task, but not in the story generation task, the control group children told longer stories. On the comprehension task, the two groups did not differ in their recall of factual information after story retelling, but the control children were better at answering story grammar comprehension questions. Merritt and Liles conclude that "while both unimpaired and language-impaired children appear to be guided in their overall story organization by the logical structures defined in story grammar, language-disordered children are less effective in their use of the grammar . . . the language-disordered children attended to the stories as well as the unimpaired children and generally remembered the details of events . . . (but) had a poorer use of their story knowledge, as reflected in their less adequate comprehension of the relationships between the story parts . . . " (p.547). This general summary of the difficulties language impaired children have with story structure fits the findings of other researchers as well (Miranda, McCabe, & Bliss, 1993; Feagans & Short, 1984; Graybeal, 1981; Gillam & Johnston, 1993; Roth & Spekman, 1985; Westby, Maggart & Van Dongen, 1984).

Assessing Children's Use of Story Frameworks

The easiest task to use when assessing a child's knowledge of story structure is story retelling. In a story retelling task, the child listens to a story, and is then asked to retell the story to a listener. Where appropriate, the child may be given the story book with the pictures intact and the print omitted to support the retelling. As Merritt and Liles (1989) discovered, and as other researchers have reported as well, when language impaired children retell stories they have listened to or read, in comparison with their language-normal peers, their stories are shorter, they use less complex language, fewer logical cohesive ties, and include less of the key information in the story. Weaver and Dickenson (1982) compared the story retelling abilities of two groups of reading-disabled children (9–12 and 13–16 years old) with the performance of a group of normal fifth grade subjects. They found that the retold stories of the reading-disabled subjects were shorter, contained more wrong information, lacked significant detail, and tended not to contain linguistic features marking temporal and causal relationships in the story. Weaver & Dickenson suggest that these results are a reflection of inefficient story processing abilities on the part of the reading disabled students, affecting both memory and comprehension systems. Naremore (1994) examined the story retelling abilities of a group of 36 children as they progressed through kindergarten, first, and second grades. She found that children who scored below average on a test of language development as kindergarteners also tended to have difficulty with story retelling. The primary difficulty was reflected in her finding that as a group, the children with low language test scores failed to retell complete episodes. In other words, the basic Initiating Event—Attempt—Consequence structure in the original story was not reflected in their retelling. The story used with the kindergarten children in this study contained five such episodes. To eliminate memory problems in the retelling task, the children were allowed to look at the pictures as they turned the pages of the book to retell the story. Many of the children in the study were able to retell four of the five episodes, and most of the children in the group whose language test scores were average retold three or more episodes. The children with low language test scores tended to include two or fewer episodes, and several of them included no complete episodes. Their story retellings sounded as though they had perceived the original story as a series of unconnected utterances.

The story used in this study was *Timothy and the Night Noises* by Jeffrey Dinardo. A summary of the story is presented below:

> *Timothy and Martin [who are pictured as frogs, but who might just as easily be pictured as little boys] are getting ready for bed. Timothy has trouble getting his pajamas on, but his mother comes and helps. After mother tucks them into bed, Timothy says he is afraid of the dark, but his mother tells him there is nothing to be afraid of, that his brother will be with him. After she turns off the light and leaves the room, Martin tells Timothy not to be a fathead. Then Timothy hears a "WOOOO," and yells for his mother, saying that he heard a ghost. She assures him that it is only the wind. She sits with him for awhile. Then he hears another noise, "CREAK, CREAK." He jumps into his mother's lap, saying, "What's that?" She assures him that it is just the rocking chair, and he rocks it himself, just to be sure. As soon as he climbs back into bed, he sees something moving on the wall. He calls for his mother, saying he sees a monster. She says it is only the shadow of a tree on the wall, and tucks him back into bed. After she leaves, Martin tells Timothy, "You're such a baby." Then the illustrations show a figure covered with a bedspread tapping Martin on the shoulder, saying "BOOO." [The reader must infer that it is Timothy.] Martin runs out of the room calling for his mother. She comes back in with him, assuring him that there is no ghost. She tucks Martin in, and turns to look at Timothy, who is fast asleep.*

Compare the two attempts to retell this story given below. The first is from an average-language child, the second from a low-language child.

Child #1

She, um, mama said he had to go to bed, so he went in there and he had trouble getting his pjs on. Then mama said, "Here you go" and he got it. The she kissed him goodnight to bed. Then he said, "I'm scared." and then she said "there's nothing to worry about it." And she closed the door and said goodnight. And they started fighting.

Then he heard a "WOOOO." And then he started calling for help and mama rushed up the stairs to the bedroom. Then he said he heard a ghost and she said "no, it's just the wind." And then she tucked him in and read the story.

And then he saw a monster. And then she came up and said, "it's nothing, it's just the tree." And then she kissed him back to bed.
And then they started fighting again and he said "I'm not scared of anything. You're a little fat head."
And then he felt something tap on his shoulder. It was BOOO, a ghost. And then he screamed for help and he got out and opened the door and called for help. And then mama tucked him back in bed but then he was, the other one was asleep. And then he said "Shhh."

Child #2
He was having trouble putting his shirt on. Turned out the light, went out the door. A ghost. A creak. She said that there's no monster and tucked him into bed. He was fast asleep. Shhhh.

This comparative example shows not only the tendency of language impaired children to give less information in their story retellings, but also the failure to indicate relationships among the events of the story, and the apparent failure to apprehend the episodic structure that makes a story a story. The second child's retelling is purely descriptive, following along with the pictures. It contains none of the episodic structure of the original story. This "description oriented" approach to the task is characteristic of children who have language problems and also of much younger normal children. (Note: The procedure we used to score these story retellings is presented in detail in Appendix 3).

Another way to investigate children's story knowledge is through spontaneous story production. Making up an original story is a difficult task—much more challenging for a child than story retelling. As Roth and Spekman (1985) point out, story construction involves formulating ideas, planning and organizing the ideas, and codifying them linguistically. Generally speaking, the younger the child, the more difficult spontaneous story production will be. Making up a story taxes every aspect of a child's expressive language ability. The child must have a meaning to convey, must be able to find the vocabulary and grammar to encode the meaning, and must also be able to call up knowledge of story structure within which to arrange the meaning. If any one part of this process overwhelms the child's abilities, the resulting story will show the effects. Research by Roth and Spekman (1985) and Westby et al. (1984) has shown that when learning disabled children or children who are poor readers are asked to generate stories which are then compared with stories told by their normally achieving peers, the results emphasize the difficulties of the story generation task. Roth and Spekman found that the stories told by the learning disabled children in their study, who were between the ages of 8 and 13 years, were significantly shorter, contained fewer complete episodes, and had less developed settings. When the episodes in their stories were analyzed, it was found that they tended to leave out the middle, or attempt, section of the episode. They also used fewer causal and simultaneity relations to tie events together. Westby et al. found similar patterns in the third, fourth, and fifth grade children in their study. The children with reading problems produced shorter, structurally simple stories with incomplete episodes. Because of the difficulty some language impaired children have with spontaneous story generation, and because retold stories are easier to score and also lend themselves to comprehension assessment, we tend to agree with Merritt and Liles (1987) that there is no substantial advantage to a story generation task over story retelling.

Why are Stories Important?

Certainly, we would like all children to be able to enjoy and learn from stories. Knowledge of story structure is a part of this ability. However, children's ability to comprehend and produce stories is related to more than their enjoyment. Research suggests a troubling set of consequences related to children's problems with stories. Recall from our discussion in Chapter 1 that Fazio, Naremore and Connell (1993) conducted a three-year longitudinal study of a group of 36 children of poverty from kindergarten through second grade. They collected a variety of measures of the children's language ability during all three of the years. At the conclusion of their study, 15 of the children were found to be in some sort of academic difficulty—ranging from being retained in grade to being required to attend remedial summer school to being declared eligible for special education services. The researchers asked whether any single measure of language ability at kindergarten might have predicted these second grade outcomes. The strongest predictor was the children's story retelling ability. Of the 15 children in academic trouble as second graders, 13 had failed the story retelling task as kindergarteners. This predictive power is not perfect, of course. Eight other children in the study failed the kindergarten story task and were not in academic trouble as second graders. Nevertheless, an inability to retell a story in a kindergarten child must serve as an alarm signal for all who are concerned with that child's progress through school. This alarm signal is all the more critical when a failure on a story retelling task is accompanied by other measures suggesting delays in syntax, low levels of vocabulary development, or difficulties in language learning in general.

Why should knowledge of story structure be so important for a child's academic progress? Perhaps because narrative discourse development has strong implications for emergent literacy in preschool children, and the ability to tell a coherent narrative predates and predicts successful adaptation to school literacy (Dickenson & McCabe, 1991;

Feagans, 1982). A child who starts to school with a knowledge of story structure has probably been read to as a preschooler, and Wells (1985), in another longitudinal study, found that the presence and awareness of print in the home of a preschooler was the best predictor of academic performance in that child as a 10 year old. Stories serve as a sort of middle ground between the interactive, context-embedded language of the home and the non-interactive, context free language of the school. Stories give most children their first introduction to what we might call "literate language," or language which is used to talk about objects, people, and events not present in the immediate context. This sort of language use, which is critical to a child's development of full literacy, will be discussed in some detail in Chapter 7. Children who have little or no experience with the language of literacy (and story retelling may be an index of such experience), or who cannot acquire it quickly upon entering school, are very likely to suffer academic failure.

SUMMARY

In summary, school aged children whose academic performance suggests that they may have difficulty with language (learning disabled children, children with reading difficulties) seem to have particular difficulty with stories. Although their literal comprehension of stories may be equivalent to that of their peers, their attempts at story retelling or spontaneous story production are marked by their shortness and lack of detail. In particular, these children seem to lack a knowledge of story structure which would enable them to construct complete episodes and to tie the episodes together using complex relational terms. The academic consequences of this lack of knowledge of story structure are becoming more evident, suggesting that intervention in the early elementary grades may be critical to the child's later academic success. In Chapter 6, we will present a case study involving three kindergarten children who cannot retell a story, along with an intervention plan for working with such children.

C H A P T E R 6

Intervention with Scripts and Stories

When we think of working with a child who is having difficulty re-counting events, or a child who is unable to comprehend or to retell a story, we are faced with a question: is the child's problem due to the absence of a framework, or to the inability to encode the framework in language? Obviously, the answer to this question will determine not only the goals we set for the child, but also what we do in intervention settings. We will consider the possibilities in the examples we give in this chapter.

GENERAL PRINCIPLES

First, let us consider the general principles that govern intervention with event recounting and stories.

1. Make sure activities use whole texts, events, and experiences.
2. Connect intervention activities to the classroom and curriculum.
3. Help the child attend to the salient features of the task.
4. Keep form, content, and use integrated in all activities.

These general principles reflect our commitment to helping the child find relevance, and to keeping language learning embedded in a communication context. They are principles that arise naturally from a sense that the most successful language intervention is that which emphasizes the whole task rather than the individual parts. As Beaumont (1992) suggests, rather than asking "How can I break this down to make it easier?" we should be asking "How can I make this more whole?" She proposes a whole-part-whole framework in which the clinician begins with a whole event, such as telling a story, singles out specific skills or parts for development, and then returns the skills to the whole in their improved or corrected form (p. 274). This whole-part-whole framework will be reflected in the case studies and the plans we give for intervention activities in this chapter.

CASE 1: MICHAEL

Tina Nelson is an experienced speech-language pathologist who has been hired to work in a new fifth-sixth-seventh grade middle school in a midwestern city. The children in her caseload are all new to her, since they come from several different elementary schools in the city. She has found that many of them have problems with writing as well as with speaking. One of the first children to come to her attention was Michael. Michael, at age 12 years, was an active, enthusiastic child whose expressive language abilities left much to be desired. He was the middle child in a family of five children, and was held back in third grade because of problems with reading. At the time the decision was made to hold him back, a full assessment was done, and Michael was determined to be language impaired. In his folder, Tina found test scores from the previous year showing that his receptive and expressive vocabulary scores were extremely low, and he had great difficulty making up sentences using relational terms such as "when" and "before." He had a performance IQ of 85, and notes from both his third and fourth grade teachers suggested that he had difficulty paying attention and staying on task in the classroom. Tina's own classroom observation revealed that Michael had difficulty staying in his seat, and seldom finished an assignment without reminders from the teacher about what he was supposed to be doing. He was frequently warned to stop talking to the children sitting around him. He answered the teacher's questions when called on, although he sometimes seemed to be guessing about what the answer should be. The most revealing information came from his response to an assignment in which the teacher asked the class to write a description of a visit they had made to a local greenhouse and plant nursery. They were told to write the description for a classmate who was in the hospital recuperating from an illness. The children worked in small groups of three, first discussing what they would say, then constructing the written narrative. The teacher put some vocabulary words on the board, and asked each group to use these words in their account. The words were: *greenhouse, nursery, transplant, humidity, temperature, fertilizer.* Michael was asked to tell about the experience in his group, while another child in his group took notes. The teacher also sat in on Michael's group to take notes. Michael's oral account was as follows:

> *Well, we went to this place with a lot of plants, and it was really hot inside because of sun coming through the glass. And they had these, like, hoses on the ceiling and they turned on the water and all the girls were like screaming and stuff. Everybody brought a plant to plant outside the window at school. And they had these rows of baby Christmas trees. We saw this big machine that moves the big trees if somebody wants to buy a big one.* [Prompt by another child: " What about Richie"]. *And oh yeah, I almost forgot, we went on Mr. Bright's bus and Richie got bubble gum on his shoe and it stuck to the floor and made a big mess. And there was this one kind of tree with long kind of stickers that would go all the way through your hand. And also there was this other plant that eats, like, flies and stuff. Gross. We got to plant some seeds in this special kind of stuff to make them grow fast, and then everybody had to wash their hands. And that's all I remember.*

After prompting by the teacher, Michael remembered that the place with the sun coming through the glass was a greenhouse, but was unable to figure out how to use the other words in his account. The teacher then took Michael aside, to work with him on a written account. He was asked to tell what should come first in the description for his classmate, and he said, "I can't remember." When prompted, he agreed that the ride on the bus must have come first, and that planting the flowers at school was the last thing, although he was unable to say why it must have happened last. His attempt to reorder the other events, using the notes taken by the teacher, was unsuccessful. Meanwhile, the other two children in his group reorganized the account as follows:

> *We took a trip to the Wilson Garden Center to visit the greenhouse and the plant nursery. We went on Mr. Bright's bus. The first accident of the day was when Richie stepped on a piece of bubble gum and got it all over the floor of the bus and all over his shoe. When we got to the Garden Center, we went to the plant nursery where they are growing different kinds of trees for people to buy and transplant in their yards. We saw pine trees, dogwood trees, and birch trees with white bark. Then we went to the greenhouse, which is made of glass so the plants can get plenty of light. There are heaters inside to keep the temperature at the right level, and there is a spray system overhead to keep the humidity at the right level and to water the plants. The second accident of the day happened when the spray came on while we were inside, and everybody*

got wet. Some of the girls screamed because their hair got wet. We saw a special collection of plants that eat insects, like the Venus flytrap. We planted seeds in little plastic pots and mixed in fertilizer to help them grow. After we washed the dirt off our hands, everybody got to choose a flower to bring back to school, and we transplanted them outside the window so everyone in the school can enjoy them.

As the group's account indicates, Michael's attempt contained some of the salient events, and also included some details which were important only to him, such as the machine used to move the larger trees. He recounted the events in no particular order, apparently as he recalled them, which is a normal thing to do at the "drafting" stage of the assignment, but then he seemed unable to come up with a strategy for reordering the events or for including the new vocabulary. His account also lacks specification of the relationships between happenings, such as why the girls screamed or why everyone had to wash their hands. Clearly, Michael's event recounting was not on a level equivalent to that of the other children in his classroom.

The first thing Tina considered about Michael's account was whether he could be expected to have a script for visiting a garden center. The answer, of course, is no. But that does not mean that he had no framework to use for recounting "trips." The framework might be viewed as a chronological one calling for specification of certain key elements. When we tell about a trip, you talk about how we travelled, and we generally proceed chronologically, picking out the events which might amuse or inform the person listening. There was no reason to assume that Michael had taken so few trips that he had no time-based framework, or that he was cognitively incapable of figuring out the causal or chronological relationships in the event. What we seem to be seeing here is a problem with encoding the event into language, and with choosing what to tell based on the probable needs of the audience rather than the interests of the speaker. Michael's generalized script structure for "trips" should serve as a help for him in organizing his account of a specific activity, if he can access it. With this in mind, Tina developed a plan for working with Michael which would embody the principles set out at the beginning of the chapter, and also would address Michael's difficulties.

Tina's overall objective for Michael was to help him encode and organize his event recountings. The specific goals and objectives were:

Goal: *Michael will use narratives to demonstrate cognitive schemata (mental frameworks) for a variety of concepts, actions, and events important for school success.*

Objective: *During script retelling Michael will link the events temporally/causally by using relational terms.*
Objective: *Michael will relate organized, coherent plans for events (eventcasts).*
Objective: Michael will use organizational strategies to communicate a script.

With her specific goals for Michael in mind, and remembering our overall intervention principles, Tina decided to do two things:

1. An Activity Outside the Classroom

Tina planned to work with Michael and three other language impaired children who had similar difficulties with event recounting. The vehicle she chose to access event recounting for these boys was a project called A Book About Our School. Specifically the boys were asked to write a book for children new to the school. It involved activities familiar to the four authors which enabled Tina to be sure that the boys had the required script and that the difficulties they experienced were in converting the script to language.

Breaking down the activity

First, Tina had a discussion with the boys about what things a new child might need to know about the school. They needed to try to take the point of view of another child, which was difficult for all of them. Tina realized that they might be helped if a hypothetical child could be described. She gave them this example:

> *David is 10 years old. He has just moved to our town. He will be coming to our school, but he is worried, because he doesn't know what the rules are, or what he should do. David is afraid he will do things wrong, and people will laugh at him. We're going to write a book for him, to help him know what to do and what not to do at our school.* She then gave the boys a few examples to help them get started. For example: *What does it mean when the bell rings twice at recess? (It means everyone should come inside immediately, usually because the weather is bad.) Did someone explain to you what it meant? (The teacher, or another child in the classroom). Do you think we might need to explain to David about this? What else happens at recess that David might not understand? If you want to play basketball, or softball, how do you get the equipment? Can you play anyplace on the playground, or are there certain places for each grade?*

In this discussion, Tina was helping the children think of the ingredients for an event that might be called recess. Other events might be *getting lunch in the cafeteria or having a fire drill or what to do if you get to the building before school starts.* Tina planned to have three or four events in the book, and she helped the children come up with ideas about which events to include, focusing always on what the hypothetical child might be confused about.

Once the children had identified likely events, Tina accompanied them on a walk-through of each event, encouraging them to talk about what was happening, and making notes as they talked. For example, when getting lunch was the focus for the day, she went with the group to the cafeteria (having previously made arrangements with teachers for all of them to go at the same time.) As they got to the cafeteria, she asked, "What's going to happen now? Can we get our food right away?" The children explained the necessity to wait in line, to pick up a tray and eating utensils, to pass by the food, telling the workers what they wanted, to choose a table, to eat, to take trays and dishes to the proper location, etc. Tina's role in this discussion was to ask leading questions, to help the children verbalize what they were doing, and to keep notes for the group. Then, after the children had walked through the event and talked about it, Tina wrote the separate pieces of the event on cards, and had the boys put them into the correct order. After a sequence had been established, they talked about "special" words the hypothetical child might need to know. The children's input was particularly valued here, since Tina realized that they had particular insights into which words might cause problems for them, or which words they regarded as out of the ordinary. They discussed whether the lunch setting should be known as the lunchroom or the cafeteria, and what to call the place where the trays were put after eating.

With the cards in order in front of them the boys were ready to write their book. Tina explained that there were important words that should be used tie a story or an explanation together. She asked the boys to try to think of any of these words themselves before introducing them. They were able to come up with *first, second, last, before,* and *after.* Tina reminded them of *while, then,* and *because.* Each word was then written on an individual card and Tina asked the boys to put them where they fit in the account. When they were in place the boys took turns reading the account. Tina asked them if the account made sense, and they made several corrections. One of the boys was a good artist, and he volunteered to illustrate each script. The other two took turns typing the manuscript into the computer.

Putting the activity back together

When the boys had finished their book, it was bound and "published," with the children's names prominently displayed on the cover as the authors. The book was placed in the school library. Each child's teacher was encouraged to have the child talk about the book, describing one event in it for the class or explaining how the book was made. This gave each boy another opportunity to practice his event recounting skills.

2. An Activity in the Classroom

Tina realized that it was essential that Michael see the importance of event recounting in the classroom. She and his teacher collaborated to find the best way to make event recounting salient for Michael. They agreed that throughout all aspects of teaching event recounting it would be important for both of them to mediate. We can not assume that Michael or any other language impaired child will understand why what we are doing is important or how it fits into his daily life in and out of the classroom. Michael's classroom teacher suggested having the children make a poster of the "words that tie sentences together" which could then be displayed for all to see. The teacher assigned a small group of children, including Michael, to work on this project. Tina served as Michael's coach during this process, asking him questions designed to help him come up with examples for using some of the words.

The art teacher also invited Tina to join Michael's class as they worked on an art project. This provided her with the opportunity to act as Michael's coach as he and his group organized their project and then later as they told the rest of the group what they did. Tina was happy to be able to work with Michael on a planning activity, since this would enable him to use language in an eventcast format. The art class had been broken into small groups, and each group was to construct a sculpture out of recycled materials such as plastic milk jugs, aluminum cans, and old lumber scraps which the art teacher had provided. Each group had to decide what they would make, which of the recycled materials they would use, and what additional supples, such as glue or nails or paint, they would need. Then they could begin by assembling the needed materials. Tina sat in with Michael's group, and told them she would be their note taker. She asked them to tell her what steps were involved in the planning process, and she wrote each step as a question at the top of a page of paper. Then, they went back and discussed the answers to the questions. Tina noticed that Michael wanted to jump from question to question, with answers about additional materials before they had resolved the issue of what they would make. She quietly coached him to stick with one question, and get the complete answer to it down before moving on to the next one. When they had finally answered all the questions, she asked Michael to be the director, reading out the plans as the other students in the group assembled the materials.

Breaking down the activity

In the long run, Tina knew she needed to give Michael (and his teacher) a set of strategies that he could use regardless of the nature of the event he was attempting to relate. She decided that teaching him to question himself before relating the event might help him organize his thoughts. This is a metalinguistic skill that was unfamiliar to Michael and to his classroom teacher as well. The sample list of questions Tina prepared for Michael is shown below:

1. Ask the question, "What kind of event is this? Is it a game? Is it a trip? Is it something I have done before?"
2. When you have classified the event, remind yourself what you know about these events. **This is the "what" and "who" step.** For example, if you are going to tell about winning the football game, what do you know about football games? Who was playing? What were the important plays in the game? What was the final score? Or, if you are going to tell about going to Disneyworld, what are the important things to tell about a trip? How did you get there? Who went with you? Where did you stay? What was the most fun? What did you hate about it? Did anything funny happen?
3. Put the happenings in the right order. **This is the "when" step.** What was the first thing that happened? What did you do after that? Then what happened? Follow this procedure until you come to the last happening.
4. Make sure you have explained the **Why** and **How** parts of the happenings. For example, why was the 30 yard pass play so important in the football game? How did you find your little brother when he got lost at Disneyworld?

These strategies were explained to Michael, and given to him on a card he could refer to when he needed to. His teacher helped him to use them in every activity that involved event recounting, including writing a book report, writing about a class field trip, and telling about something he did on the weekend. Tina worked with Michael outside the classroom to help him apply the strategies, and she and the teacher both worked as coaches when Michael had an assignment. The role of the coach was to help Michael remember what he had been taught about strategies, and to help him put the specifics of the event he was recounting onto the framework provided by the strategies. Strategy teaching is a highly metalinguistic activity, and not all language impaired children are able to use their metalinguistic abilities to organize their thinking. Helping Michael to do this was an important part of intervention at his level, and it took some time for him to use the strategies without coaching.

SCRIPTING ON A DIFFERENT LEVEL: CASE 2: KERRY

Kerry was a kindergarten child who was diagnosed as language impaired when he was four years old. He had two years of intervention before he began school, and he was enrolled in a kindergarten class at age six. His receptive language was within normal limits, as tested by the CELF-Preschool. However, his expressive language abilities did not reflect what he seemed to know about language. This is an example of a child whose test scores were unrevealing of his actual language use in communication. His CELF-Preschool expressive score was only one standard deviation below the mean, but when Frank Barnes, his school speech-language pathologist, collected a language sample, he observed that Kerry's syntax and morphology became quite immature when he attempted to engage in connected discourse. His response to "Tell me what happens when you go to school" is given below:

> Well, we write and we read and we go outside. One day we hided from the teacher and she just was, she just called and called, and we comed. And one day we could go to the auditorium to see a magic, a man with magic tricks. And he asked to, if, he wanted somebody to help him, and Don raisded up his hand, and he said what your name is and all like that.
> But what happens in your class? What do you do in class? What's the first thing you do in the morning?
> We read, and we write.
> Is that what you do first?
> Yeah. Well, sometimes we have free time and the teacher says you could play or make stuff.
> And then what happens?
> We just keep on, and we do that some more and some more.

Compare this account with the account below, taken from a study by Robyn Fivush (1984) in which language normal kindergarten children were asked the same question:

> "I turn over my name. I do my handwriting. If I have time, I do my art project. Then we have meeting time. Then we have math time. Then we

have another meeting with snack. Then sharing, if it's Friday. If not, story with snack. And sharing if it's Friday. After snack and story, mini-gym. Go to the bathroom, have lunch, then you get a little play time. And then we have Ron's [science class] or nap" (p. 1709).

Fivush summarizes the results of her study as follows: "All children tended to mention those acts that occupied a particular time and place in the classroom, and each of these acts seemed to encompass a list of possible activities in a hierarchic fashion . . . These results indicate that children represent an event as a general spatial-temporal framework based on the first experience with a new routine; this framework becomes more elaborate and the temporal and the hierarchical organization of the representation becomes more complex with increasing experience with the event" (p. 1697). In contrast to the children in Fivush's study, Kerry seems not to be using a script. He recalled some unique events which had stuck in his memory, but he did not respond with a temporally or hierarchically organized account of the school day. Frank observed Kerry in the classroom, to find out whether he seemed disoriented or confused about the routine. He observed that, far from seeming confused, Kerry often anticipated what would happen next, and he even protested when the teacher attempted to replace the regular story time with a music lesson. What could Kerry's problem be?

SCRIPTING VS. SEQUENCING

Many of our students, when confronted with a child like Kerry, tell us at once that they will work with him on sequencing. Our response is always, "Why?" Kerry is not confused in the context of the classroom. He knows what happens there. Showing him sequences of picture cards about planting flowers or putting out fires and asking him to put them in the right order is not likely to have any effect at all on his ability to recount what should be a scripted activity. Going back to sequencing might be appropriate for a preschool child who is genuinely confused about the ordering of events, or about the meaning of first or last. Kerry's problem is on a different level. His immature verb morphology on this task (he made only two morphological errors on the CELF-Preschool) and his frequent false starts suggest that the task is a difficult one, which taxes his language abilities. If he could learn to use his existing script as a framework for his account, he would find the task less taxing. With this in mind, Frank designed a classroom based intervention activity.

An Activity in the Classroom

Goal: *Kerry will verbalize his scripted knowledge of common events.*

Working within the event

Kerry, like other language impaired children, will find it easier to use language within the context he is talking about than removed from the context. Frank enlisted the help of Kerry's teacher in appointing a "reporter" for each day. The job of the reporter was to remind the teacher and the other children in the class what would happen at each transition point in the day. So, when the children assembled in the classroom, the teacher would turn to the day's reporter and ask, "What will we do first this morning?" Three other children had this job before Kerry was appointed. On his day, Frank asked the teacher to take notes of what he said, and these notes were turned over to Frank, who put each event mentioned by Kerry on a separate note card. One day, Frank took a Polaroid camera into the classroom and asked the teacher to take photographs of the children as they engaged in the various events of the day.

Taking the event apart

All the children in Kerry's class had activity time in the classroom every day, during which they were allowed to work in one of the activity centers in the room. There was a nature center, a book center, and, most importantly, a writing center. Frank came into the classroom twice a week to work with Kerry at the writing center, where he proposed that they should make a book for the class reporter to use to help organize the day. Frank showed Kerry the note cards, with simple phrases such as "story time" and "snack time" on them. On each note card, Frank had glued the appropriate picture of the class. He agreed to type the words for the book if Kerry would help put them in order. Together, they agreed on the order for the cards, and Frank went away to type them. The next time he came in, he brought the typed account, which he had purposely disorganized. He began the day with rest time and recess, followed by snack time. He explained that he had accidentally dropped the cards, but that he thought he had everything right. Kerry and two other children, who had spontaneously joined them at the writing center, corrected him. They found the scrambled account so funny that Frank decided to put it in the book along with the corrected account. But this time, he sat at the computer with Kerry at his shoulder to tell him what to say. Although Kerry had not begun to read, he was given the re-ordered note cards with the pictures and words on them to use as cues, and he gave Frank an organized account of the day.

Putting the event back together

Kerry and Frank decided to call their book "A Silly Day at School". The book told the story of a space creature who tried to go to kindergarten and was asked to be the reporter for a day. He got everything confused, and the class had to make him sit in the corner while they told him how the day really was. They illustrated it with a picture of the alien drawn by Kerry and with the Polaroid photographs of the children in Kerry's class engaged in their routine activities. Frank and Kerry read it together several times, and then engaged in a joint reading for the class. It quickly became the most popular book in the room, in part because it had everyone's picture in it, and in part because the children found it so funny.

Some notes about this activity

Kerry is a language impaired kindergartener who has not begun to read. Why, then, are we using printed note cards and making a book for him to "read"? This is not carelessness on our part. Kerry must become a reader. He needs to learn what print can do. He needs to begin to feel comfortable with it. This is important for all school-aged children, particularly those who are language impaired and likely to have problems with reading. We used book writing with Michael, the older child in the first case study, for similar reasons. For children Michael's age, who have had many negative experiences with print and reading, producing a book of their own can be an exciting event.

Another thing to note about the activity with Kerry is that it takes place entirely in the classroom, within the regular daily activity. It is an example of good collaboration between the speech-language pathologist and the teacher. The teacher is not asked to spend extra time doing some lengthy new activity. She can integrate an activity designed to help Kerry into her regular routine, involving other children as well. The SLP works within the regular schedule of the room as well, so Kerry is never pulled out, and never misses anything that happens in the class. While this may not always be possible, it is possible much more often than it is practiced. It takes a little creative cooperation between teacher and SLP.

Some notes about assessment

The assessment information given for Kerry was not made up out of our heads. He is a real child. It is important to note that, when given the CELF-Preschool, he did not score like a language impaired child. His impairment only became apparent when he was asked to use his language knowledge in the service of communication. When he had to organize and structure language above the word and sentence level, his morphology and syntax began to sound like that of a much younger child, and he showed evidence of how difficult this task was for him. This simply underlines the remarks we made in Chapter 1 about the inadequacy of standardized tests for assessing the language problems of school aged children.

One final note is in reference to the language used to attempt to elicit scripts from children. As we pointed out in Chapter 5, it is important to ask a question which will encourage a child to give a general account, not a memory of some specific day. Such questions as "Tell me what you did at school today" or "Tell me about school" are not likely to be effective with language impaired children. The question used in our elicitation, "Tell me what happens when you go to school" was used by Fivush (1984) in her research, and we used it in order to be able to compare Kerry's account with the accounts given by the children in the study. It is a carefully phrased question, in that it does not refer to a particular day or time, but rather focuses on the school experience as a gestalt.

CASE 3: AARON, MIKE, AND JOSH: WORKING WITH STORIES

Katie Moore, a school speech-language pathologist, works in a large urban elementary school with a student body made up almost exclusively of white children from poverty. Some of these children are bused in from adjacent rural areas, and some are city children whose parents are without employment and on welfare. Many of the children in her caseload have suffered from inadequate medical care, and some have been abused or neglected. Every spring, she meets with the kindergarten teachers in the school to discuss those children who are at risk for failure as they enter first grade. Katie and these teachers have worked together for several years, and she has explained to them the language behaviors she considers good signs of possible trouble. She has come to trust their instincts as, year after year, their referrals more often than not turn out to be children who do have language problems. Last spring, one teacher referred three boys: Aaron, Mike, and Josh. She said that all three were having great difficulty with phonics, and seemed generally unprepared to function in the classroom environment. At the beginning of the fall, Katie asked the school psychologist to do a nonverbal IQ test (the *Columbia Mental Maturity Scale*) with each boy, just to give some indication of whether they needed to do full scale evaluation. She also administered the TOLD-2P, collected a conversation sample, did some metalinguistic testing, and a story retelling task. Some of the data from this evaluation are presented below:

Mike was 7 years, 2 months old at the time of the testing. His non-verbal IQ was 94. On the metalinguistic tasks (presented in Appendix 3), he was able to recognize only three of 12 ungrammatical sentences, and he could not correct what was wrong on even those three. Phonological awareness was poor, in that he was unable to do any of the phonological elision tasks and could do none of the metalinguistic word segmentation tasks. In conversation, he was able to talk with Katie about his new baby brother for five turns, but then shifted topic, with no marking of the shift, to talk about playing soccer after school. On the TOLD-2P, he scored 1 standard deviation below the mean on picture vocabulary and oral vocabulary; 2 standard deviations below the mean on grammatical understanding and grammatical completion; and 1.5 standard deviations below the mean on grammatical completion. On the story retelling task, he was unable to retell any complete episode out of the five in the story. His story retelling is presented below. (A summary of the story is presented in Chapter 5, and the scoring procedure used can be found in Appendix 3.)

Putting on their clothes. He's walking. Mother is kissing them. There's nothing to be afraid of. He jumped on his mother's thing. A tree. There's nothing at the window. Tapped him on the shoulder.

Aaron was 6 years, 7 months old at the time of the testing. His non-verbal IQ was 80. The metalinguistic testing showed that he could recognize nine of the 12 ungrammatical sentences, and correct seven of them. Phonological awareness was poor, however, He was able to do only 30% of the phonological elision tasks, and only 40% of word segmentation tasks. His conversation was lively, marked by frequent topic shifts which he marked by asking questions. On the TOLD-2P, he scored 1 standard deviation below the mean on grammatical understanding and sentence imitation; all other subtests were within normal limits. On the story retelling task, he was unable to retell any complete episode of the five contained in the story. His retelling is presented below:

They went to bed. Mom. Then he tried to put on his nightgown and he couldn't. So his mom put it on. Then she tucked him in bed. And she gave him a kiss in the head. And he hears a noise. And he said "Martin is in there to protect you." And turned off the lights. And she ran out. And Martin said "You're so a wimp." WOOO. It was just the wind. So she tucked him back to bed and told him a story and kissed him on the head again. And he heard a cricket. And it was just a rocking chair. And he saw something on the wall. And it was just a tree. So she tucked him back in. So she tapped on the hand and Timothy . . . And it was a ghost. He jumped out of bed and ran out the door. And he was fast asleep.

Josh was 7 years, 6 months old at the time of the testing. His non-verbal IQ was 90. Metalinguistic testing showed that he was able to recognize seven of the ungrammatical sentences, and to correct five of them. His phonological awareness was poor. He seemed unable to comprehend the phonological elision task, and was able to get only 50% of the word segmentation items correct. He was noticeably reticent in conversation with Katie, giving one or two word responses to all her questions, and he initiated no topics on his own. On the TOLD-2P, he scored 1 standard deviation below the mean on oral vocabulary. All other subtests were within normal limits. On the story retelling task, he was unable to retell any complete episode of the five contained in the story. His retelling is presented below: (Note: "ahhh" is our representation of a scream.)

He's going to bed. He's having troubles. They are both getting kissed but he goes "AHHH!" Don't turn out the lights. His mom's going out the door. He hears "WOOOO" sound. Then he thinks it's a monster. Then it's a creak, creak, creak. It's just the rocking chair and it goes creak. It's the tree again, ahh it's a monster, it's just a tree shadow. Ahhh, it's the cover. Help me, help me, ahhh, help. Shhhh, don't let nobody know.

Katie decided to work with the three boys in a group, even though their story retelling and underlying language skills looked rather different on the surface.

She noted that even the child with the least amount of story structure (Mike) managed to include some elements of the setting, or beginning, and the ending. Aaron, whose retelling was most complete, usually retold an initiating event and a consequence for an episode, and told parts of four of the five episodes in the story. Mike had some setting statements, but no pattern in what he chose to retell. He got a piece of three of the five episodes, but his story retelling was extremely sketchy. Josh also had some setting statements, with no pattern in which parts of an episode he retold. He seemed to have one part of all five episodes, but sometimes he had an initiating event, sometimes an attempt, and sometimes a consequence.

Katie decided to focus her intervention efforts on the episode structure itself. She knew that an understanding of story structure would help the students derive meaning from the story and would facilitate their recall and prediction abilities as well. The goals and objectives she set for the group were as follows:

> **Long Term Goal:** *Each child will demonstrate a conscious awareness of episodic structure and will use this awareness to analyze and construct stories.*
>
> **Objective:** *The student will become familiar with story structure and the language used to talk about stories by participating in read-aloud sessions on a daily basis.*
>
> **Objective:** *The student will use language to verbally relate the "problem" of a story.*
>
> **Objective:** *The student will use language to verbally relate "problem-attempt" relationships within stories.*
>
> **Objective:** *The student will use language to verbally relate "story outcomes."*
>
> "**Objective:** *The student will retell complete episodes in stories.*
>
> **Objective:** *The student will incorporate at least one complete episode in an original story.*

1. An Activity Outside the Classroom

Katie's first action was to have a meeting with the boys' teacher, to explain what she would be working on, and to encourage the teacher to use the same terminology about stories that she would be using. They agreed that the classroom teacher would focus on identifying "problems," both in stories and in everyday classroom events. Katie decided that she would begin by doing a series of mini-lessons with the three boys on episodes. Then she and the teacher would provide a similar lesson for the entire class.

Working within the event

Katie began by having a discussion with the boys about problems. She defined a problem as "something that is hard to deal with," and gave them several examples of her own, such as having a flat tire in a rainstorm, or locking her office door with her key inside. They immediately began to discuss problems they had encountered, or that people they knew had encountered. When she was certain they had a firm grasp of problems, she mentioned that every story contains a problem, and encouraged them to listen for the problem in the story she would read to them. She then read *Mouse Soup* by Arnold Lobel.

Taking the event apart

After she read the story, Katie asked the boys to talk with each other, and decide what the problem was in the story. While they talked, she prepared a visual organizer to help them with story structure, like the one shown in Figure 6-1.

When the boys reported to her what the problem was, she wrote it into the appropriate box on the chart, and put the chart on the bulletin board. (Note: the clinician should continue to work on identifying problems in stories until the children are able to find these without undue difficulty. This may take one or several sessions, depending on the children.)

When the boys came for their next session, she reminded them of their discussion about problems, and said "When we have a problem, we always have to figure out how we're going to solve the problem. When I had a flat tire in the rain, I had to figure out how to get the tire changed without getting wet. So I stopped at a service station and let them change the tire while I waited inside. When I locked my keys in my office, I had to find Mr. Winston (the custodian) and get him to let me in with his keys. Let's talk for awhile about how we solve problems." The boys were encouraged to discuss solutions to problems, some of which involved much more violence than Katie had expected (many problems were solved by killing or shooting someone). However, she decided to save the discussion of peaceful solutions for another time, recognizing that the concept of solving a problem was one the children could deal with. Once again, she took out *Mouse Soup* and asked the boys to listen for the solution to the problem they had written on the chart previously. After her reading, they discussed the solution together, and agreed what she should write in the chart. (Note: this focus on solving problems should continue until the children can find the solution in a story context without undue difficulty. The problem-solution link should always be presented in a story, although a part of a longer story might also be used.)

In her third session, Katie reminded the boys that sometimes, when you try to solve a problem, your attempt works, and sometimes it doesn't. She said:

Every time you try to find a problem, there is an outcome. The outcome might be good, or it might not be. But it's always there. For example, when

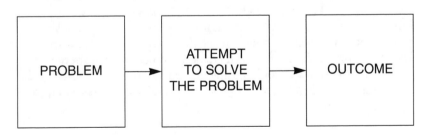

Figure 6–1. A visual organizer for story episodes.

I had the flat tire in the rain, I solved it by pulling into a service station. But if the service station had been closed, the outcome would have been bad. When I locked my keys in to office, I tried to find Mr. Winston. I found him, and he was able to let me in. That was a good outcome. Let's talk about outcomes now. Your teacher told me that you had a problem with the guinea pig in class this week. What happened? [He got out of his cage.] And how did you try to solve the problem? [Everyone stood on the other side of the room, so nobody would accidentally step on him, and the teacher picked him up.] And what was the outcome? How did this end? [The guinea pig went back in his cage and went to sleep.] Right. Every story has an outcome. Let's read Mouse Soup *again, and look for the outcome.*

After her reading, the boys discussed the outcome, and it was entered onto the chart. (Again, this focus on outcomes should continue until the children are able to identify them.) At this point, she introduced the term "episode," and explained that whenever they found a problem, a solution, and an outcome together, these would be called an episode.

In the fourth session, Katie chose a new book, one that had a simple problem-solution-outcome structure, but had more than a single episode. She explained to the boys before she began that sometimes a story might have more than one episode, but that they should still look for problems, solutions, and outcomes. She chose to read *The King, The Mice, and The Cheese* by Eric and Nancy Gurney. After the reading, she went back to the beginning of the story, and asked the boys to help her find the first problem, followed by the first solution, followed by the first outcome. Each episode was entered onto a chart, until they had the entire story divided into episodes.

Putting the event back together

When the children had filled in the chart for the book, Katie gave the book to Aaron and asked him to tell the story, making sure he got all the episodes. She told him he could use the pictures to remind him what happened in the book. She chose Aaron because his initial story retelling had been best, and she believed he would be able to retell the story. After returning to the whole event with Aaron, she continued to read stories to the boys, which they would analyze together, and each boy took a turn to retell the story. With Mike and Josh, she tried to stay with books having few episodes and obvious structure, to make the task less daunting for them. She even encouraged collaborative retelling in the beginning, so they would be able to recreate the story. Some of the books Katie found are listed in Appendix 4, with some notes about their episodic structure.

2. An Activity in the Classroom

After Katie had taught Aaron, Mike, and Josh about episodes, but while she was still working with them on story analysis, she and the teacher presented a lesson about episodes to the entire class. After reading the book *Jason's Bus Ride* by Harriet Ziefert to the class, Katie and the teacher discussed the problem, the attempts to solve it, and the solution. (Note: depending on the children's level of story knowledge and the amount of exposure they have had to stories, this might be done in three sessions, with one devoted to problems, one to solutions, and one to outcomes). They introduced the children to the term "episode," and then announced that they were going to help the children write their own stories. The class was divided into two groups, one working with Katie and one with the teacher. Each child was given three pieces of paper and crayons. First, they talked as a group about problems, and every child was told to think of a problem they might have, or someone else might have. Many examples were given, and then the children were told to draw a picture of a problem on one piece of their paper. When the pictures were complete, Katie and the teacher wrote on the bottom of the picture a sentence about the problem, such as "Rachel's mother has lost her wallet." The children then discussed how the problems might be solved. Again, many examples were given, and each child was asked to choose a solution to the problem, and draw a picture of it. The teacher and Katie wrote sentences on the bottom of each picture, such as "Rachel and her brother looked everywhere for their mother's wallet." Then outcomes were discussed, and outcome pictures were drawn and labels were written, such as "Rachel found the wallet under the car seat." The children then took turns "reading" their stories to those in the other group, and also took the stapled together book home to read to their parents. (Note: this picture drawing might be done in three separate sessions in the classroom, if necessary. Some children take a long time to draw pictures, and this might be a time consuming activity.)

Some Notes About These Activities

The key aspects of the activities given above are these:

1. Always work with real stories, preferably those found in books, so the children will have exposure not only to stories but also to print.
2. Remember that in attempting to make story structure obvious to the children, and to teach them the words to talk about it, you are working on a metalinguistic level. That is, you are using language to talk

about a language event (stories). This is cognitively difficult for some children, and it might be necessary to proceed slowly.

3. When putting events back together, strive to put the child in an active role, as a story reteller or story author. Children need to use language to tell and retell stories just as much as they need to use language to talk about story structure.

SUMMARY

The goals and objectives we have given for the children we talk about in this chapter are, of course, designed for these children. However, they are typical of the sorts of goals and objectives we might expect to find in an IEP for any child having difficulty with scripts or stories. The activities we used were, of course, designed for these children and these goals. Again, our activities are typical of the sorts of activities one might use to help children meet the stated goals. It is worth recapitulating our general principles here:

1. Make sure activities use whole texts, events, and experiences.
2. Connect intervention activities to the classroom and curriculum.
3. Help the child attend to the salient features of the task.
4. Keep form, content, and use integrated in all activities.

Adhering to these principles will challenge the creativity of any speech-language pathologist, but we believe it will result in real change. Real change is that change which carries over from the therapy setting to the child's everyday life in the classroom or on the playground. And that is, after all, what we all want for every language impaired child with whom we work.

C H A P T E R 7

"I Can't Write and I Hate to Read": Text and the Encounter with Literacy

In this chapter, we will discuss that aspect of school which is, for many language impaired children, the most frustrating and failure-laden: the introduction of reading and writing. Even those language impaired children who have begun to use language to converse with their peers and to recount their experiences and ideas orally may falter when they encounter text. This chapter will consider the reasons why that happens, leading up to a discussion in Chapter 8 of how to intervene. We will begin our discussion of text by introducing the case of Melanie.

Melanie is 8 years old and has just begun third grade. She has not been successful in school to this point, and she is not looking forward to the new year. As a second grader, she scored in the third percentile on reading comprehension on the state-mandated achievement test, and in the twelfth percentile for math. These low scores meant that she was required to attend summer school to prepare for third grade. She hated it, and does not believe that her reading improved at all. By her own report, she does not like to read, and hates to write even more. Melanie has also been classified "communication impaired," and has been receiving language intervention from Karen French, the school speech-language pathologist, since midway through her first grade year. Her spontaneous expressive language has improved remarkably over the past eighteen months, and in casual conversation, she sounds like other children her age. Karen French has just completed her beginning-of-the-year assessment of Melanie's language, however, and the results of this are not so encouraging. These results are reported below:

Story retelling: Karen read the story *Pookins Gets Her Way* by Helen Lester to Melanie, and asked her to retell it. The story has six episodes, and Melanie was able to retell only the first of them. After that, her retelling consisted of descriptions of the pictures in the book. These results suggest that Melanie was not using a story framework to structure her story retelling, which discouraged Karen, since she had worked with Melanie on episodic frameworks throughout the second grade. She reflected, as she often did, that children with language impairments did not seem to benefit from summer vacations. Karen also gave Melanie the CELF-R, primarily because she was interested in finding out how Melanie would do with the formulated sentences and sentence assembly subtests, which had caused her great difficulty the year before. She discovered that Melanie's scores on those two subtests were 2 standard deviations below the mean, but that she scored at or near the mean on the word classes, word associations, and recalling sentences subtests. Karen also collected a conversation sample with Melanie, both to check her topic initiation and maintenance skills, and also to elicit some scripted event accounts. She asked Melanie to tell her about a trip her family had taken to Florida over the Labor Day weekend, and they talked about their mutual dislike of fishing with slimy worms. Karen discovered that Melanie gave a relatively well-organized, interesting account of the family's trip to Florida, and that she was able to initiate new topics smoothly, at one point even relating the new topic to the old one. Karen also noticed that Melanie's sentence structures in this conversation were all quite simple, and the only words she used to tie together the sentences in her account were "and" or "and then."

Karen has asked for a conference with the Chapter I reading teacher and Melanie's third grade teacher. She thinks it might be time for her to shift her attention to written language, but before doing so, she wants to find out what kinds of demands will be made on Melanie in her third grade classroom, and what kinds of support she will be getting elsewhere.

ORAL AND WRITTEN LANGUAGE: THE UNRESOLVED RELATIONSHIP

Let us leave Karen and Melanie for a while, and examine some of the information that will undoubtedly play a role in Karen's decisions about how to help Melanie. We know that Melanie's oral language performance is below par for her age. We also know that she is having difficulty with reading. What is the relationship between these two aspects of language? Do language impaired children always have problems with reading and writing? Is reading difficulty a symptom of language impairment? Can we predict what sorts of reading problems a child might have, based on what we know about the child's oral language abilities? There is a growing body of research in the field of communication disorders bearing on these questions. We will summarize the results of this research under three headings: what is the relationship between oral and written language, what can we predict about a child's reading or writing performance from knowledge about oral language performance, and what specific characteristics of text might be expected to cause problems for language impaired children.

WHAT DOES TALKING HAVE TO DO WITH READING AND WRITING?

There are several options one must consider when answering this question. The first, and most obvious, is that there may be no relationship at all. Many speech-language pathologists have acted as though this were the case by insisting that their only concern was with what came out the child's mouth and what went into the child's ears. The idea that print on a page is "language," and that the child's comprehension of this language, and the child's ability to express ideas in this language might derive from spoken language abilities, seems foreign to these professionals. Indeed, if reading is seen primarily as a visual skill, and writing is seen as a matter of spelling and letter formation, such attitudes make a great deal of sense. This is a point of view which would define reading as essentially that process we call "decoding"—figuring out which letters make which sounds, and putting the sounds together to make words. The assumption seems to be that if a child can do this, then the child can read. Unfortunately, the child's ability to assign meaning to the words, sentences, and paragraphs of a text once the words have been decoded is ignored, or taken for granted. If one views writing as the physical act of forming letters on a page, with spelling as a corollary, then certainly the speech-language pathologist may quite reasonably insist that a child's writing ability is something someone else should deal with. The idea that a child may have difficulty finding the words to express meanings, or organizing those meanings into coherent texts, is apparently ignored, or taken for granted. In short, we would agree that for a child whose oral language skills are normal, reading or writing difficulties are probably not the business of the speech-language pathologist. But a child who has had difficulty acquiring language in the preschool years, and whose oral language abilities are delayed will almost certainly have difficulty with reading and writing, even if decoding is not itself a problem (and this is a big "if"). This child's problems with meaning and organization are certainly the business of the speech-language pathologist, just as are meaning and organization in spoken language.

A second option to consider when asking about the relationship between oral and written language is that oral language forms the foundation for written language—that reading and writing are somehow "grafted" onto listening and speaking. There is, of course, some sense in which this is true. Assuming that a child is functioning in a monolingual situation, the child is reading and writing the same language she speaks and hears. The vocabulary and the grammar will be familiar. If the child can speak and understand a sentence like "The girls jumped over the stream," then, decoding problems aside, the child should be able to read and comprehend or to write this sentence. If one adopts this point of view, then it would be logical to say that a child who was having trouble with reading should be given help with listening comprehension, and a child having difficulty with writing should be given help with oral expression. The assumption is that when the oral language base is in good shape, then reading and writing will be natural, easy processes for the child, assuming the presence of normal visual and fine motor abilities. This viewpoint ignores the anecdotal evidence provided by many parents and teachers of children who are having trouble with reading: their spontaneous spoken language does not suggest that they are language delayed or language disordered. In fact, some of these children do fairly well with reading as long as they are allowed to read material they themselves have dictated. One approach to teaching reading, sometimes called the "language experience" approach, capitalizes on this ability by teaching children to read their own language, written down by the teacher. This approach allows a child to build on his own set of meanings and his own vocabulary, concentrating on problems of decoding alone in the beginning. After the child has become a fluent decoder of his own language, then the words and ideas of other writers may be introduced. While the language experience approach to reading has much to recommend it, and undoubtedly does play to the child's strengths, every child must eventually be able to read more than what he is able to construct himself. And it is at this point that many children begin to experience difficulty. This is the point at which we must begin to recognize that much of what children read is more than "spoken language written down." Oral and written language are not exactly alike, and this fact leads to the third option for thinking about the relationship between them.

The third possibility, and the one we find most persuasive, is that oral and written language exist in a symbiotic relationship. For the preliterate child, and the child who is just beginning to read and write, oral language is predominant and indeed forms the basis for reading and writing. For the literate child, however, written language influences and flows into spoken language, not only in terms of ideas and concepts, but also in terms of vocabulary and syntax. Most accomplished readers and writers have a "reading" vocabulary that they acquired from books, not from speaking. This vocabulary is available to us when we speak and listen, however, as well as when we read and write. This same sort of learning applies to certain complex sentence patterns, which are seldom used in casual conversation, but are often seen in writing. Such familiar patterns as the "not only/but also" structure are examples of this. These patterns are made familiar to us from the printed page, and eventually find their way into our spoken language. But beyond this, the nature of written language compels us to master ways of signalling organization that we never use when we talk. What is the spoken equivalent of a paragraph, for example? How often in conversation with friends do you find yourself using summaries, or telling your listener how many points you will make in a particular argument? Written and oral language are indeed symbiotic, but there are some important differences—differences which will have significant consequences for language impaired children. We will now turn our attention to these.

Text and talking

To understand the primary differences between text and talking, we need first to think about the context in which children acquire language. It is a context of talk—specifically, a conversational context. As we learned in Chapter 3, one of the key characteristics of conversation is negotiated meaning, that process by which conversationalists combine and build upon individual meanings to come up with a meaning greater than (or at least different from) what any one of them might have expressed alone. Consider the building and negotiating in this conversation among a group of first graders about the concept of "charity."

A. It's when you have to help people, like if they're real old or something.
B. Sometimes if people get sick and they have to get medicine and stuff and they don't have any money.
C. It's when people don't have anyplace to live, and they're homeless, and you give them money and stuff.
A. But people are poor and they still have houses, like in the TV show Mrs. Flynn showed us.
C. Yeah, but maybe they have roofs that leak and their windows are all broken and in the wintertime they don't have any way to get warm.

B. _Yeah, and they can go to the Salvation Army or someplace like that and get coats and gloves and stuff._

A. _And you're supposed to help other people if they're poor or sick or homeless and they need medicine and stuff._

None of these children alone could give a clear-cut definition of "charity," and yet they manage to come up with a pretty clear sense of it, working together. Children are accustomed to negotiating meaning in this way from the time they first learn to talk. Adults do it as well. It is a hallmark of conversation. However, it is not a skill that serves us very well when we are faced with the necessity to construct a meaning using only our own language, with little or no shared experience to depend on. This is what we must do when we construct text.

Text is not interactive, and it is not based on shared context. Written language (and some oral language, such as classroom lectures) exists not as a series of utterances spoken in alternating conversational dialogue, but as a monologue. The reader does not have the contributions of other speakers to build on when constructing meaning as a conversationalist does. Meanings in written language exist as relations between utterances (cued by words such as "therefore" and "on the other hand") and as inferences to be made from arguments or from sequential ideas. Meanings are not negotiated; they are carried by the language of the writer. There are no gestures, facial expressions, or vocal changes to signal changes in focus or approach. There is no opportunity to stop the speaker and ask for clarification. Clarification may be provided in the written text by the use of paraphrase, redundancy, and examples. Both the writer and the reader must come to recognize these conventions, and know what is signalled by phrases such as "in other words" or "for example." Text uses language and a special set of linguistic conventions to establish meaning.

Wallach and Miller (1988, p. 84) express the differences between oral interaction and reading as follows:

> Readers must engage in several levels of processing at once: they must hold in mind questions to determine if the actual text answers them, and if so, how, when, and where; they must marshal their own experiences and knowledge as a counter-argument to the author's; they must withhold those of their own experiences that do not pertain to what is being proposed . . . Finally, readers "must have learned to negotiate the world of abstractions" (Postman, 1985, p. 26). Negotiating the world of abstractions involves an understanding of and an ability to manipulate decontextualized ideas divested of whatever concrete images they might have held.

As this statement suggests, the transition to literacy for children involves more than a switch from using their ears to using their eyes.

Written language is not just spoken language on paper. Becoming literate involves new cognitive processes as it opens up a world of language beyond interaction.

These new cognitive processes are demanded by three aspects of textual language, and they are discussed in the following pages. They are not total departures from ways of thinking children have done before, and yet they do involve some abilities to manipulate language and meaning that are unprecedented in most preliterate children's language use. In particular, three new ways of approaching language and deriving meaning from language, arising from the demands of textual language, will cause difficulties for language impaired children when they encounter literacy. They are **metalinguistic knowledge, cohesion**, and **inferencing.**

METALINGUISTIC KNOWLEDGE

Do you remember when you first began to study grammar in school? Probably it involved the "parts of speech," and you were required to find all the adverbs or all the participles in a given paragraph of text. Many students find this sort of exercise quite difficult, and frustrated teachers often ask, "how can you speak a language and not be able to analyze it?" There is a great difference, of course, in the tacit knowledge we have of our language which allows us to speak and understand automatically, and the kind of knowledge we must have to analyze the language. The latter is called "metalinguistic" knowledge, and it involves using language to talk about or think about language. In effect, for most of us, language is like the glass in a window. We know it is there, but we are too busy looking through it to be aware of it. If we have to, however, we can make ourselves look at the glass rather than *through* it. We do this when we have to decide whether the glass is dirty, for example. In a sense, when we are using our metalinguistic knowledge, we are looking at language rather than through it. We are holding language as an object of perception. We make multiword sentences all the time, without thinking about how many words each sentence contains. If necessary, however, we can think about how many words we're using, and can make a sentence exactly seven words long, or follow the instructions to "make a twelve word sentence using the word "more." When we do this sort of task, we are using our metalinguistic knowledge, which allows us to count the number of words in a sentence and to be aware of using a specific word.

Children's metalinguistic knowledge develops over time. Two-year-olds may spontaneously correct their own utterances when they are aware that what they said didn't sound "right", showing an awareness of how utterances should sound which is separate from meaning. Preschoolers as young as 3 years of age may play with rhyming, making up strings of nonsense words while laughing at their own silliness. Sometimes a 4 year old might say "I can't think of the right word" or "what does that word mean?" suggesting that they are aware of word as an entity. Beyond these sorts of behaviors, however, most preschool children show little metalinguistic awareness. In fact, many preschoolers have difficulty separating a word from its meaning, as one 4 year old showed when asked to "tell me a long word." His answer was "mile." When asked why that was a long word, he replied "because it's a long way." Researchers generally agree that while metalinguistic awareness may appear early in some children's development, it continues to develop throughout the early elementary grades. and most children achieve some workable level by age 7 or 8 years (Saywitz & Cherry-Wilkinson, 1982; Kamhi, 1987).

Several factors appear to govern the appearance of metalinguistic awareness in children. Metalinguistic awareness may be related to the child's cognitive development, particularly the development of centration, which allows the child to hold and manipulate two ideas in the mind simultaneously. It is centration abilities which allow children to concentrate on both height and width when judging the size of a figure, for example, or to be aware of both meaning and syntactic form when judging the appropriateness of an utterance. Many kindergarten children demonstrate the beginnings of centration, and most children show it by age 8 years.

In addition to its cognitive underpinnings, metalinguistic awareness seems also to be related to how much a child has learned about language in general. Cazden (1974) suggests that children must be able to produce and comprehend a particular linguistic form for some time before they are able to make judgments about its correctness. The exact level of primary language abilities necessary for metalinguistic abilities to be manifested is unclear, however. Perhaps the best summary of this relationship for normally developing children is van Kleek's (1982), "Clearly metalinguistic skill requires some primary language competence, if only because the child must have something to reflect upon " (p. 256). For language impaired children, however, the relation between primary linguistic ability and metalinguistic ability is somewhat less clear. Kamhi and Koenig (1985) found that language impaired elementary school children had great difficulty making explicit judgments about language form, such as whether a given sentence was correct or incorrect. They report that these children were generally able to comprehend and produce the syntactic forms they had difficulty judging, but this did not ensure that the children would be able to make a judgment about appropriate use of the forms. They speculated that the language impaired children's representations of syntactic forms might not be as well established or as stable as those of normal children. The reasoning here is that language impaired children will have difficulty reflecting on and manipulating the same kinds of information and knowledge that they have difficulty encoding and learning.

Metalinguistic abilities also seem to be related to a child's IQ and can be affected by environmental stimulation. Bright children whose parents play rhyming and word games with them will show more met-alinguistic awareness than slower children whose environments never involve such language play. Perhaps less obviously, the presence and use of print in a child's home will also play a role in the environmental stim-ulation of metalinguistic abilities. As Miller (1990) points out:

> Children in high-print homes have multiple opportunities to interact with language. They are encouraged to talk about language, about talking, and about listening . . . . language is something that is considered and observed both orally and in print . . . . the oral and print language users in the home apprentice children into language through directing the chil-dren's attention toward such things as the humor resident in linguistic ambiguity and toward the special relationship between words and their referents . . . . Within the context of a high-print home, children typically develop an understanding that language is something that can be manip-ulated, transformed, made up, and written down. (p. 15)

The implications for children from less stimulating environments, with less advanced cognitive skills are clear: their metalinguistic skills will be delayed compared with those of more fortunate children. This may have particularly unfortunate results when they encounter reading instruction.

Why is metalinguistic knowledge related to reading? As Wallach (1990) points out, the sounds of speech are more or less continuous, while print on a page is broken into units separated by white spaces. A child who is beginning to read must figure out how individual letters and words on a page represent the continuous sound that they hear coming out of their own and other people's mouths. "Young readers must become linguists. They must bring their spoken language knowl-edge to the surface and develop a more analytical sense about language and its parts. Beginning reading is the time when the implicit becomes explicit and the linguistic becomes metalinguistic" (p. 65). Several researchers (Wallach & Miller, 1988; Blachman, 1984; Bradley & Bryant, 1983) have shown that children who begin the reading process with some knowledge of word, syllable, and sound boundaries are better read-ers. Tunmer and Nesdale (1985) point out that children who have a sense of syntactic and sound segments of language recognize that print reflects certain structural features of spoken language earlier than children who do not. In particular, they emphasize the importance of phonological and structural awareness.

Phonological awareness has been suggested by many researchers to be a prerequisite for success in learning to read (Golinkoff, 1978; Bradley & Bryant, 1985; Wagner & Torgeson, 1987; Catts, 1989). In order to learn to decode words, the child must be able to do more than produce the sounds that correspond to each letter. The child must be aware that speech comprises phonemic units and be able to analyze and synthesize the units. As Nesdale, Herriman, and Tunmer (1984) point out, "Knowing the phonemic units in the spoken word, the child is then able when confronted with the printed word, to map the latter onto the former." Most children require formal instruction to master skills associated with phonemic awareness. However, it seems that children who demonstrate some phonological awareness upon entering school will most readily benefit from beginning reading instruction. But presuming that all young children have a rudimentary awareness of phonemic units and basing instruction on such an assumption, will certainly contribute to the difficulties some children experience.

Van Kleek and Bryant (1984) report examples of phonological awareness in the language of some children as young as 2 years of age. For example, one 2 year old reported spontaneously that *witch, watch,* and *water* all began with the same sound. Undoubtedly, children from high-print homes whose parents foster such awareness may demonstrate it quite early. However, the results from experimental data suggest that many children of school age cannot consistently demonstrate phonological awareness. A variety of experimental tasks has been used, such as counting segments, breaking words into constituent sounds, and identifying initial or final sounds. Van Kleek and Schuele (1987) suggest that "preschool children's lack of success on these tasks may have been a result of the nature of the task (i.e., drawing on the abstract basis of the phoneme) as well as the type and number of operations to be made on the word (e.g., segmentation, synthesis, elision)" (p. 27). Generally speaking, children seem to have an easier time identifying initial than final sounds, and both of these tasks are easier than segmenting a word into all of its constituent phonemes.

Because children are unlikely to know the word "phoneme," and because they tend to think instinctively of syllables when asked to divide a word into parts, Fox and Routh (1975) simplified the segmentation task by asking 3-, 4-, and 5-year-old children to tell "a little bit" of a word. For example, the examiner would say "bed" and ask the child to say "a little bit of it." If the child responded with "ed," the experimenter then asked the child to say "a little bit" of "ed." The task enabled the child to divide the word into syllables, and the syllables into phonemes. Generally speaking, they found that the children's performance improved with age, with 3 year olds able to segment only about one fourth of the syllables into phonemes. Other studies, such as those by Zhurova (1973) and Smith & Tager-Flusberg (1982) developed novel and entertaining ways for children to demonstrate phonological awareness, and found that 3 and 4 year olds have only minimal success with such tasks. If some normally developing children have difficulty with phonological awareness, what can be said about language impaired children's ability?

While we have known for some time that language impaired children are likely to have problems learning to read, it has sometimes been difficult to say exactly why. Studies have reported significant correlations between measures of semantic-syntactic language abilities and later reading achievement (Tallal, Curtiss, & Kaplan, 1989; Bishop & Adams, 1990). An even larger body of research has consistently indicated a strong relationship between early word recognition and phonological awareness, however (Bradley & Bryant, 1985; Fox & Routh, 1983; Liberman & Shankweiler, 1985; Lundberg, Olofsson, & Wall, 1980; Tunmer & Nesdale, 1985). To give only a few examples of the findings from such research involving language impaired children, consider the following. In 1990 a study conducted by Magnusson and Naucler found that the best predictors of reading achievement in first grade for language impaired children were measures of phonological awareness. The abilities to make rhyme judgments and to identify phonemes in words were found to be closely related to reading outcome in their language impaired subjects. Similar results have been reported by Menyuk et al. (1991), who studied 130 children at risk for reading disabilities and found that measures of metalinguistic abilities, including phonological awareness, were the best predictors of reading achievement. Catts (1993) identified a group of 56 children with language impairments in kindergarten, and measured a variety of speech and language behaviors including phonological awareness. Subjects were followed in first and second grades and were given tests of reading achievement, including measures of written word recognition and reading comprehension. He found that many of these language impaired children fell behind their normal-language peers on measures of word recognition in first and second grades and on a measure of reading comprehension in second grade. Examination of his individual subject data showed that approximately half of the language impaired subjects were reading within normal limits in first and second grades, whereas the other half were not. In an attempt to account for those children who had trouble reading versus those who did not, Catts looked at the speech and language abilities of the children. He found that when reading was assessed in terms of word recognition, both in isolation and in context, measures of phonological awareness and rapid naming proved to be the best predictors of reading outcome. Reading comprehension, however, was more closely related to measures of semantic-syntactic language abilities than to phonological awareness. In fact, results indicated that after semantic-syntactic measures had been partialed out of the analysis, phonological awareness measures accounted for none of the variance in reading comprehension.

To summarize the importance of metalinguistic awareness as it relates to reading in language impaired children: reading comprehension is based in a child's overall language competence, including the child's knowledge of vocabulary and syntax. Decoding, however, is probably more clearly related to metalinguistic knowledge. If a child is being taught to read using a phonics approach, phonological awareness is a critical component of the reading process. As a child progresses from simple decoding of words to more complex reading tasks, such as finding the main idea, morphological and syntactic awareness become necessary (Tunmer & Bowey, 1984). As van Kleek and Schuele (1987) put it, "These types of awareness engender segmentation and synthesis skills, which the child uses to segment sentences into words and words into phonemes, as well as to synthesize phonemes into words." (p.20). This suggests that any kindergarten child known to be language impaired should be assessed for phonological awareness, and that any kindergarten or first grade child who is experiencing difficulty with phonics should be similarly assessed. Teaching phonological awareness to children at this stage can help to prevent long-term problems with reading, and the associated academic failure experienced by far too many children.

INFERENCING

To understand the importance of inferencing to literacy, it is necessary to return to a discussion of the nature of text. In a text, meaning exists not only in what is said, but also in what the reader or listener brings to what is said. Consider the following:

> *The men dug into the bunker as sniper fire was heard to the west. They wondered when their reinforcements would arrive.*
> *Who are these men and in what event are they participating?*

> *Jim slipped into his aisle seat just as the musicians began to tune their intruments. He opened his program to find out what the first number would be.*
> *Where is Jim and what is about to happen?*

*Janet drank her orange juice while waiting for the bacon to cook. Mary
made toast and looked for the cereal.
What time of day is it?*

All of us can answer the questions above, in spite of the fact that the
answers are not given in the brief text preceding the questions. We can
answer the questions because, as experienced readers, we automatically
bring to bear our knowledge of the world as we read. This act of using
prior experience and knowledge of the world to interpret what we read is
called constructive comprehension or **inferencing**. Inferencing is a
process of constructing associations and making things fit together
which is a natural part of assigning meaning. It is such an automatic
process that we are often not even aware of doing it. Research with adults
shows that we often cannot separate information we inferred when reading a story from information which was actually given in the text (Ackerman, 1986; Klein-Konigsberg, 1984). Children also make inferences
when reading or listening to stories. Children as young as 6 years of age
infer information, and they become better at constructive comprehension as they progress through the early elementary school grades.

Much of our information about language impaired children's inferencing abilities has come from research published in the past decade. Of
particular importance is the work of Ellis Weismer (1985), Crais and
Chapman (1987) and Bishop and Adams (1992). These studies have been
organized around a series of questions about the comprehension abilities of language impaired children: Are children's story comprehension
abilities predictable from standardized language comprehension scores?
Do language impaired children perform more poorly on comprehension
questions requiring inferencing than on questions requiring literal
recall? Do language impaired children perform better when inferencing
from stories presented pictorially than from stories presented verbally?
and finally, Is there an identifiable subset of language impaired children
who perform worse on inferencing tasks than other groups of children
who are also language impaired? Ellis Weismer studied 12 seven- and
eight-year old language impaired children, Crais and Chapman had 16
nine- and ten-year-old language impaired subjects, and Bishop and
Adams studied 61 8- to 12-year old language impaired children. The
results of these three studies were in general agreement. First, in all
these studies the language impaired children's story comprehension
was at a level equivalent to that of language normal children two to
three years younger. Second, the children's story comprehension abilities are poor regardless of whether they are asked for factual recall or for
inferencing. And finally, the children perform as poorly with pictorially
presented stories as they do with verbally presented ones. These results
will be discussed below, along with one additional finding on which the

studies disagree: Ellis Weismer found that her subjects did as poorly on a standardized comprehension test (the NSST) as they did on the story comprehension. Bishop and Adams, on the other hand, found that story comprehension scores were worse than scores on a comprehension test (the TROG).

Before turning to the points of agreement among the studies, let us discuss the disagreement. Bishop and Adams (1992) suggest that one explanation for the discrepancy in the findings might be statistical in nature. That is, because they had more subjects in their study, their statistical comparisons are more powerful. Assuming that this is the case, and that the results of the Bishop and Adams study are an accurate reflection of language impaired children's comprehension abilities, why might we expect story comprehension to be harder for these children than comprehension of items on a standardized test? These results are more likely to be understandable if we consider the nature of standardized tests of language comprehension. These tests are designed to assess children's understanding of syntactic and morphological contrasts, and the child is usually given a choice of four pictures, one of which exemplifies the contrast. For example, the item to which the child is responding might be "Show me 'The man has eaten'." The pictures show a man with a full plate of food in front of him, a man in the process of eating, with the plate half full, a man watching while another person puts a plate of food onto the table, and a man looking down at an empty plate and smiling. The child is given visual support (by looking at the pictures) and is only called upon to deal with meaning conveyed within a single sentence. While many language impaired children have difficulty even with this kind of comprehension task, the comprehension of stories is not analogous. As Bishop and Adams explain, story comprehension demands constructive processing. The reader or listener must establish a context within which to interpret the information. Inferencing is what allows us to establish the contexts which govern our recall and our comprehension. Without inferring a context, we will be forced to interpret a story as a series of unconnected utterances, and all the meaning which exists between the lines will be lost on us. The failure to construct a context will make it extremely difficult for us to answer the first question we all ask about a story: "What is this story about?" In the words of Bishop and Adams, "understanding of connected text requires constructive processing by the reader or listener, rather than just passive reception. One could therefore argue that SLI children do poorly on story comprehension because they do not engage adequately in such constructive processing. In contrast, they do relatively well on TROG, in which understanding of literal meaning is tested for sentences presented one at a time" (p. 35).

This failure to engage in constructive processing explains another result found in studies of language impaired children's inferencing: language impaired children not only perform poorly on questions asking for inferences, they also perform poorly on questions about factual details of the stories. Such failures cannot be attributed to memory deficits on the part of these children, because they show the same deficiencies when responding to questions about picture stories even with the pictures visible to them. The more likely explanation is that constructive comprehension, or inferencing, provides the child with a framework for a story, and all aspects of the story are understood and remembered within this framework. As Oakhill (1984) expresses it, "skilled comprehenders are more likely to use relevant general knowledge to make sense of information implied in a text, and . . . such inferential and constructive processing helps not only their understanding but also their literal memory for the text" (p. 36). It is not entirely clear why language impaired children fail to engage in constructive processing. It is possible that they simply lack sufficient world knowledge, either because they have limited experience or because they fail to store or retrieve memories of that experience. It is also possible that these children have the experience, and have the memory of it, but are unable to apply it in relevant situations because of some cognitive or processing limitation.

Imagine, for example, a language impaired child who has had a normal amount of experience with being afraid in the dark, or imagining monsters in the closet or under the bed. The child has just read or listened to the story *There's a Nightmare in My Closet* by Mercer Mayer, about a little boy who frightens the monster in his closet and makes it cry, and eventually puts it into his bed to comfort it. A child who is a skilled comprehender will immediately put him or herself in the place of the boy in the story, and will project various other ways to frighten the monster and also will be able to talk about how the monster feels, why it cries, and what the boy might do if another monster appears. The language impaired child, on the other hand, is likely to have difficulty recalling factual details provided in the story (such as what the boy said to make the monster cry) as well as projecting or making inferences about the general situation of being afraid of monsters. One possible explanation for this failure is that the child is unable to retrieve from memory his or her own experiences of being afraid of the dark, or is unable to retrieve them in a form which makes it possible to relate them to the story. If this were the case, one might assume that prompting the child to recall previous experience, and asking questions designed to prompt applying this experience to the story might help the child. It is also possible that this child does not see that his or her own experience of being afraid of the dark is relevant here, and so treats this story as a unique and new bit of information about the world. This would seem to imply some difficulty with grouping or categorizing experiences, some lack of abstract or overriding concepts on which such groupings might be made. If this explanation is accurate, one might expect to see evidence of difficulty with categorizing in other encounters with text, such as finding the main idea of a paragraph. One might also expect to see performance improve if the child were given the principle on which the grouping should be made, such as "think about being afraid of the dark" or "think about what to do if you see a monster." Or, it is possible that the child is simply incapable of making any sense at all of the text, and so has no idea what experiences in his own life it might relate to. This seems unlikely unless the vocabulary and sentence structure of the text are outside the child's existing language knowledge. Without further research, we cannot be certain about the causes of the language impaired child's failure to apply existing knowledge to the task of comprehending text.

Some attempt to explain the source of the problem is found in Ellis Weismer's (1985) explanation for the finding (shared by Bishop and Adams (1992)) that language impaired children had as much difficulty comprehending stories presented in pictures as they did comprehending stories presented in words. Both Ellis Weismer and Bishop and Adams report this finding as being perhaps the most unexpected in their studies. While admitting that this finding might reflect the fact that inference construction depends to some extent on verbal mediation regardless of the mode in which material is presented, Ellis Weismer says,

> It is possible to speculate that deficits in aspects of imagery or mental representation may hinder language-disordered children from effectively abstracting and generating links between relevant pieces of information in order to integrate that information in a meaningful fashion. In terms of language comprehension, this would mean that even when language-disordered children understand individual words or sentences, they tend not to 'read between the lines' as readily as their age mate to arrive at a full understanding of the message (p. 183).

In other words, with some support from previous research (Johnston & Ellis Weismer, 1983; Savich, 1980; Kamhi, Catts, Koenig, & Lewis, 1984), she is arguing that language impaired children have what she calls "islands of deficits in other cognitive processes related to inference construction."

Finally, the question of whether there is some identifiable subgroup of language impaired children who have problems with inferencing was asked by Bishop and Adams (1985). This question is relevant because previous work by these authors and others (Rapin & Allen, 1983; Bishop & Rosenbloom, 1987; Rapin, 1987) suggests that there is a group of language impaired children whose problems are not with grammar or sentence formation but rather with language content and use. Such children have been described as "over literal," focusing exclusively on the surface structure of sentences in a conversation, for example, and failing to comprehend intended meanings. Although many clinicians can report having seen and worked with such children, and George, the child whose conversation is analyzed in Chapter 3 of this book seems very much like the children Bishop and Adams (1989) describe, the results of the Bishop and Adams (1992) investigation do not support the hypothesis that such children might have particular problems with inferencing. On the contrary, all the language impaired children found story comprehension difficult.

What, then, does this body of research suggest about reading problems and language impaired children? It seems fair to say that, even when decoding or reading accuracy is not a problem, reading comprehension may be problematical for language impaired children. As Bishop and Adams (1992) put it, ". . . . the current study suggests that reading comprehension failure can arise from children's difficulties in integrating information within a story and using general knowledge to deduce what is not explicitly stated" (p. 127). This suggests, in turn, that teaching language impaired children strategies to help them bring their real world knowledge to bear on texts may have important consequences for the child's academic performance.

COHESION

Another aspect of text which may be problematical for language impaired children is **cohesion**, which involves how meanings are tied together in a text. Mentis and Prutting (1987) point out that "cohesion is achieved through the linguistic interdependence of elements within a text" (p. 88). Cohesion arises at any point in a text where the meaning of some aspect of text can only be determined by reference to information contained somewhere else in the text (Blank & Marquis, 1987; Mentis & Prutting, 1987). A coherent text can be seen as a unit in which the parts are tied together by various kinds of meaning relations. These meaning relations are signalled by the use of what Halliday and Hasan (1976) have called **cohesive devices.** Table 7-1 provides a list of the five kinds of meaning relations identified by Halliday and Hasan,

TABLE 7–1. Cohesive ties.

Relation	Example
Referential	*Mary* likes candy. *She* eats *it* every day.
Lexical	Some *animals* are dangerous. *Lions and tigers* are particularly fierce *creatures.*
Substitution	Last night I *learned to tango.* I never thought I'd be able *to do that.*
Ellipsis	I'm going to study tonight. *Are you?*
Conjunction	Phil played golf *after* he mowed the lawn. *Before that,* he had painted the porch.

together with examples of the cohesive ties used to signal these meanings. These five major meaning types are: referential, lexical, substitution, ellipsis, and conjunction.

The following brief text, which has been pulled apart with the sentences numbered for ease of analysis, provides examples of all five types of cohesion:

1. *Last night I dreamed I went to Hawaii on vacation.*
2. *I have always wanted to* **do that.**
3. *Everything* **there** *was green and beautiful.*
4. **It** *was like I imagine the Garden of Eden must have been .*
5. *In my* **dream***, there were very few people in* **this paradise.**
6. **On the other hand***, there seemed to be more aninmals than I ever saw in one place before.*
7. *There must have been at least one of every kind of* **creature** *on earth.*
8. *Don't ask me how* **they** *all managed to live together without eating* **each other** *up.*
9. *I have no idea.*
10. *But they* **did.**

Reference is used to tie together *Hawaii* and *there* in sentences 1 and 3, and *Hawaii* and *it* in sentences 1 and 4, and *creature* and *they* in sentences 7 and 8. Lexical cohesion makes the tie between *Hawaii* and *this paradise* in sentences 1 and 5, and *I dreamed* and *in my dream* in sentences 1 and 5, and *animals* and *creature* in sentences 6 and 7. Conjunction can be seen in sentence 6, in the form of *on the other hand*. Substitution is used in sentence 2, where *do that* substitutes for *went to Hawaii on vacation*. Ellipsis can be seen in the last sentence, in which *did* signals the omission of the phrase *live together without eating each other up.*

As this brief example suggests, even the shortest sample of text will be filled with cohesive devices. When do children learn to use cohesion, and what are the earliest devices found in their language? Even 2-year-old children have been found to use reiteration of noun phrases and pronouns to achieve coherence in stories (Bennett-Kastor,1983). Probably the earliest cohesion attempt is repetition, in which a child simply repeats all or part of a previous turn. Stoel-Gammon and Hedberg (1984) suggest that referential and lexical cohesion appear first in children's language, followed by conjunction, substitution, and ellipsis. Liles (1985) points out that "use of cohesion as described by Halliday and Hasan (1976) is fairly stable by age 6. . . .even cohesive adequacy is fairly stable by age 7:6" (p. 28). The use of cohesive devices is obviously constrained by the child's linguistic knowledge as well as by the child's understanding of narrative conventions. However, several researchers (Bennett-Kastor, 1983; Karmiloff-Smith, 1980; Bamberg, 1987) have suggested that there is a big developmental change around age 5 years, when children become significantly better at using cohesive devices to tie together the sentences in a narrative. As Liles (1993) summarizes this change, "The observation that intersentential coherence appears to accelerate at the approximate age of 5 years is consistent with investigations of content structure and semantic use. This observation has led some researchers to suggest that there is a global reorganization at this point in development and that there is some qualitative change in how the child perceives and reports narrative organization" (p. 876).

Liles (1993) goes on to point out, however, that the development of cohesive abilities does not plateau at age 5 years. Ripich and Griffith (1988) studied the coherence in story retellings by children between the ages of 9 and 12 years. They found that the number of cohesive devices used increased as the children's age increased, and that older children made fewer reference errors. Bamberg (1987) analyzed children's stories told in response to a wordless picture book. Anaphoric pronoun use and nominal reference changed with age (up to age 10). Bamberg also found that even the 10 year olds failed to approximate adult strategies.

Unfortunately, our knowledge of language impaired children's use and comprehension of cohesion is limited. Liles and her colleagues (Liles, 1985; 1987; Purcell & Liles, 1992) have conducted several investigations with language impaired and language normal school age children. Their results indicate that, between the ages of 7 and 10 years, language impaired children's manner of cohesive organization and the adequacy of cohesive ties in their narratives differs from that of language normal children. In general, the language impaired children used fewer reference ties than their language normal peers, and had more difficulty keeping their narratives coherent. They showed the same tendency to self-correct cohesive meanings when necessary, but their attempts to correct were less adequate. Because narrative comprehension results from a complex interplay of background knowledge, schema knowledge (see Chapter 5), and linguistic knowledge, it is difficult to generalize about the effects of any one aspect of text on comprehension. However, as Wiig and Semel (1976) point out, many school-aged language impaired children have difficulty with relational terms, such as "before" and "during." It is possible, then, that some cohesive devices, particularly conjunctions, may not be part of language impaired children's vocabularies. When this possibility is combined with other aspects of text comprehension, Westby's (1984) summary is understandable:

> Whatever the nature of learning-disabled students' difficulty on narrative tasks, all learning-disabled students exhibit greater difficulty with literate than oral language skills. Although their oral language abilities may not be commensurate with other students their age, their literate language skills are even more delayed and frequently become proportionately more delayed as they continue through the educational system. (p. 121)

SUMMARY

Let us return now to the case of Melanie, presented at the beginning of this chapter. Karen French has conducted some informal assessment, designed to find out about Melanie's metalinguistic knowledge, her comprehension of cohesive devices, and her inferencing abilities. (The specific items used by Karen in the assessment described here are presented in Appendix 3.) Karen took her metalinguistic assessment items from the research by Kamhi and Catts (1986), asking Melanie to engage in sentence segmentation, phonological elision, phonological segmentation, and morphological judgment. She found that Melanie had few problems with the phonological elision task, making only two errors when asked to delete both the initial and the final sound from monosyllabic words. For example, when she asked Melanie to "say the word 'prince' with the 'p' left off," Melanie said "in." Karen was careful to make sure Melanie understood the task before she began, and she gave her the sound, not the name of the letter, when asking her to delete a sound. Melanie performed less well on the sentence segmentation task, on which she was asked first to repeat a sentence which Karen said, and then to say "a little bit" of the sentence until she could no longer divide it. Melanie could divide two and three word sentences into the individual words, but when the sentences got longer, she was never able to get to the individual word level with her segmentations. On the morpheme judgment task, Melanie was asked to judge the accuracy of 16 sentences, 12 of which contained morphological errors (such as "I tried get the book"). She was also asked to correct any sentence she judged to be "not good." Melanie was able to tell that 10 of the 12 incorrect sentences were not good, but she was able to correct only 5 of them. To assess Melanie's understanding of cohesive terms, Karen asked Melanie questions about some sections of text they read together. She found that Melanie often failed to comprehend pronoun reference, particularly "this," "that," "these," and "it." In addition, Melanie seemed not to understand conjunctions expressing causal and consequence relations. Karen used the procedures suggested by Bishop and Adams (1992) to check Melanie's inferencing abilities. She also made up some items herself, using second grade textbooks. She discovered that Melanie had particular problems with cause-effect inferences and feeling-attitude inferences. Having this information gave Karen some ideas about targets for intervention with Melanie, and she decided to make some time to sit down with Melanie's teacher to go over the assessment she had done and explain where she believed Melanie might be having the most difficulty. In Chapter 8, we will discuss Karen's intervention plan for Melanie, along with some suggestions she made to the teacher for classroom activities to strengthen all the children's understanding of cohesion and inferencing.

CHAPTER 8

Intervention for Children Who Have Problems with Text

Children who have difficulty with text are at a great disadvantage in the classroom, particularly as they move out of first and second grade and into third grade, where what they learn is increasingly presented to them in the form of written text. Many language impaired children, who have made progress in producing and comprehending speech by the time they are 8 or 9 years old, are confronted with academic failure due to their inability to handle the demands of written language. As we pointed out in Chapter 7, spoken and written language are quite different. Just as the language impaired child was slow to develop spoken language, and needed help learning to use many aspects of the spoken language system, so also this child will be slow to learn the conventions of written language, and will need extra help to develop strategies for comprehending and producing text.

In this chapter, we will first deal with the case of a child who has problems with phonological awareness. We will then return to the case of Melanie, introduced in Chapter 7, and develop an intervention plan to help her and other children like her. We will discuss strategies for helping children identify cohesion, for developing inferential abilities, and for finding the main idea of a text. Our intervention approach will be characterized by a focus on meaningful text, and by a belief that our goal must be to help the language impaired child develop strategies to use in any encounter with text. We will use the child's own textbooks as the textual material in our intervention lessons, and we will supplement these with trade books related to the curriculum topics being covered in the classroom. As we pointed out in Chapter 2, using a Social Studies or Science textbook in language intervention does not mean that we plan to teach the content of those subjects. We are not functioning as tutors. What it does mean is that we will use content important to the child as the "raw material" to which the child must learn to apply the text strategies we will teach. In addition, our intervention will involve careful mediation. Feuerstein (1979) defines mediated learning as an interactional process between the developing child and an adult, in which the adult mediates the world to the child by "framing, selecting, focusing, and feeding back environmental experiences" to produce "appropriate learning sets and habits" (p. 179). When serving as a mediator, the speech-language pathologist is not so much giving a child information as helping the child to focus on key elements of a task, scaffolding to help the child achieve success. The framing part of mediation is frequently omitted when we work with children, making it extremely difficult for a language impaired child to establish a meaningful context for what we are doing. We will present some fairly detailed examples of mediation in this chapter, to show what we mean by this.

As we did in previous chapters, we will present intervention strategies in the context of case studies. In addition to Melanie, the child you met in Chapter 7, who needs to work on cohesion, inferencing, and main idea, you will meet Ray, a first grade child in Karen French's caseload, who needs to work on phonological awareness. We will begin by presenting the goals and objectives we decided to work on with Ray, and then we will present a series of teaching activities designed to help him with phonological awareness.

CASE 1: RAY—WORKING WITH METALINGUISTIC AWARENESS

As we pointed out in Chapter 7, there does appear to be a subset of language impaired children who have not developed phonological awareness by age 6 years. Because phonological awareness is so necessary if the child is being taught to read using phonics, and because reading difficulties have such serious consequences for the child throughout the rest of school, we believe that intervention in this area is one of the most important activities a school speech-language pathologist can engage in with kindergarten and first grade children. Obviously, if a child cannot decode the words in a text, there will be little possibility for him to comprehend it! Since phonological awareness is so important for the decoding enterprise, we turn to the case of Ray, another student in Karen French's caseload. Ray was referred by his first grade teacher midway through the year, because he was having so much trouble with reading. He was unable to decode more than a few words, and he seemed baffled by the task of "sounding out" words he didn't know, in spite of a full year of phonics instruction in kindergarten. Ray was referred for a full psycho-educational evaluation, to determine whether he needed special education services and if so, what sort. The reading specialist attempted to evaluate his reading using pre-primer materials, and she found that his decoding performance on even these low-level texts was well below average. His first grade teacher reported that he seemed not to have "caught on" to phonics at all. Karen French went first to observe Ray in the classroom. She noted that he was well-behaved, and participated in all classroom routines. He followed the teacher's directions without difficulty, and seemed particularly to enjoy art and music activities. However, when it was time for reading, which the teacher conducted with small groups of children gathered in a corner of the classroom, Ray became a different child. He resisted going to the reading corner, and when he finally did get there, he squirmed around in his chair, was never on the right page in his book, and responded to all questions with "I don't know." Karen concluded that he was well aware of his reading problems, and that he was attempting to avoid this activity. She decided to evaluate his story retelling abilities, his event recounting abilities, and his phonological awareness. Not to her surprise, she found that he could not retell any complete episodes in the story she read to him, in contrast to other first grade children who could tell more than half of the episodes in the story. She asked him to tell her about a trip his class had taken to a local dairy, and found his account extremely brief and disorganized. His only cohesive tie in the account was the word "and," and he violated the chronological sequence of events when telling about the trip. For the phonological awareness assessment, Ray was asked to do phonological elision (If you take the "p" off the word "pin", what will be left?), to count the phonemes in real and nonsense words (Put down one of these blocks for every sound in the word "hi".), and to segment words into phonemes (What is the first sound in the word "fan?"). Ray was unsuccessful on all of these tasks. Karen observed that he appeared to be randomly guessing, acting as though he had no idea what he was being asked to do.

In the case conference, Ray was determined to be communication impaired. His performance IQ was within normal limits, but his performance on the language tasks was well below that of other children his age. It was clear that his language abilities, particularly his lack of phonological awareness, would have a negative impact on his academic performance. Ray was eligible for the Chapter I reading program, and

Karen and the Chapter I teacher discussed the possibility of doing some work together using trade books to help Ray become aware of episodic structure in stories. Karen began immediately to work with him outside the classroom on phonological awareness, using the three step plan developed by Ball and Blachman (1991) and Blachman, Ball, Black, and Tangel (1991). As Blachman (1991) describes it, in each lesson there is a phoneme segmentation activity called "say-it-and-move-it," followed by one of several segmentation-related activities. The final step involves games designed to teach letter names and sounds. Karen began her work with Ray by mediating for him. She explained that they would be working on words and sounds, to help him with his reading. She also told him that he already knew a lot about words and sounds, and that he would be able to use what he knew in the activities they would do together. She worked with Ray twice a week, and each session consisted of three phases. In the first phase, Karen put a small pile of blocks on the table between herself and Ray. Then she put in front of him a blank piece of paper. She instructed him to move one block off the table onto the paper for each sound in the target word. She began with single phonemes, moved to two-phoneme words, and finally to three-phoneme words. For example, one session went as follows:

> *Ray, we're going to do our sound exercises now. Here are the blocks, and here is the paper we'll put the blocks on. Remember, you will move one block for every sound in the word. I'll do the first one, then it will be your turn. Ready? Here goes. Show me /a/.* Karen prolonged the sound, and as she said it, she moved one block from the table to the paper. Then she said *Ok, it's your turn. Ready? Show me /i/. You say the sound with me while you move the block.* Again, she prolonged the sound, encouraging Ray to do the same while he moved a block onto the paper. After five single-sound items, they moved to two-phoneme words, such as "in," "at," and "up." Karen modeled the first item, saying the word slowly, prolonging the first sound, moving one block for the vowel sound and another block when she shifted to the final consonant sound. Again, she asked Ray to repeat the words with her while he moved the blocks on succeeding turns. After five items, they moved to three phoneme words such as "sun," "fan," and "leaf." Karen modeled the first one, moving a block every time she changed to a new sound. The words were pronounced slowly, with each sound being prolonged. Ray repeated the words with Karen as he moved blocks during his turns.

Following this activity, Karen and Ray moved to the second step, which involved helping Ray to hear the similarities in sounds found in different words. They might do rhyming games, or they might try to think of all the words they could beginning with the sound "s." Sound blending activities were also used in this part of the lesson. Karen would say a word one phoneme at a time, such as /b/ /i/ /t/, and Ray would get a token if he could tell her what the "real" word was. After five tokens, he received a sticker.

In the third segment of each session, Karen and Ray worked on letter names and letter sounds. Karen developed a set of picture cards for each letter of the alphabet. The B card had boys batting balls. The K card had kids kissing kittens. In the beginning of each session, they would choose five sounds to work on, and Karen would hold up each card and say the letter and the words associated with it. Following this, Karen might hold up a card with only the letter on it, and ask Ray to find a matching card from among five she placed in front of him, and then to tell her the letter and the sound. Or they might play a version of the card game "go fish," taking turns asking for letters, and responding with the sounds as they passed the cards to each other. Eventually, Karen used Scrabble tiles and she and Ray would take turns spelling three letter words for each other which they would then have to pronounce. Nonsense words were allowed in this game, so long as they were correctly pronounced. Every intervention session contained one of each of the three kinds of activities described here. In addition, Karen took time to read a book with Ray in every session, usually one of the Dr. Suess books focusing on sounds, such as *Hop on Pop* or *The Cat in the Hat.* She wanted Ray to have extra exposure to print, and to have some fun with sound as well.

These activities, and many others described by Blachman (1991) were designed to be used with groups of children in the classroom, and could certainly be used as classroom activities by collaborating teachers and speech-language pathologists. They could also be used by the speech-language pathologist working alone with a small group of children. Blachman reports that the activities are useful even when the groups are heterogeneous. She says, "Although children need to understand the concept of one-to-one correspondence to represent one sound with one disk, children in the group may vary greatly in their knowledge of letter names and sounds and in their awareness of the phonological segments in words. Within the structure of the group, it is possible to give some children a two-phoneme word to segment with blank tiles, whereas others are comfortable segmenting three-phoneme items with letter tiles" (p. 58).

CASE 2: MELANIE—WORKING WITH COHESION, INFERENCING, AND MAIN IDEA

We will return now to the case of Melanie, who was introduced in Chapter 7. Melanie's reading problems are not related to phonological awareness. Her decoding skills are considerably better than her comprehension skills. In addition, Melanie's writing skills reflect the same sorts of problems with text that are seen in her reading comprehension. We will be addressing both comprehension and production problems in the pages which follow.

Goals and Objectives for Textual Cohesion

Goal: Melanie will use and understand cohesive devices to increase logical construction and comprehension of text.
Objectives:
Melanie will use specific strategies to identify cohesive ties in text.
Melanie will identify lexical ties used as cohesive devices.
Melanie will identify substitution ties used as cohesive devices.
Melanie will identify lists of supporting information related to the main idea of a text.
Melanie will use cohesive ties in her own writing samples.

Activities for teaching

Teaching about cohesion involves some activities familiar to all speech-language pathologists, in that it essentially consists of helping the child with new vocabulary and with reference, including pronominal reference. We did some forecasting of this teaching in Chapter 6 when we talked about teaching "words that tie things together." In that case, we were helping the child use these words in his own scripted event accounts. In the current case, we will be helping the child to recognize cohesion in printed text material and use it in her own writing. It is well to be aware, when working with the child's textbooks in this area, that graded text material may not contain many of the cohesive devices we are accustomed to as adults. The two paragraphs below, the first from a third grade and the second from a sixth grade Social Studies book, will serve as examples of how the language used in textbooks changes from grade to grade.

1. *"But we have many endangered animals in our own country. The Alaskan brown bear, spotted leopard, and whooping crane are but **a few. Some of these** animals have become endangered because of too much hunting. **Others** are dying because of land development. **As** people clear the land for houses, the **animals'** food supply is destroyed. **Still other animals** are being poisoned by air and water pollution"* (Joyce & Erickson, 1991, pp. 276–277).

2. *"Many species and breeds of animals are disappearing at the present time. **Some disappear** because of uncontrolled hunting and fishing.*

*Other animals die because the habitat in which **they** had lived was destroyed. **As** the human population on earth increases, more and more land is cleared to make room for homes, farms, industries, and transportation. **When** habitats are gone, **animals die out**. Pollutions of the water, soil, and air by chemicals are **also** causes of **animal deaths**"* (Elbow & Greenfield, 1991, p. 104).

We have marked the cohesive devices in each passage, and classified them below.

1. **a few** — word substitution, referring back to "endangered animals" in line 1, signalling ellipsis (the whole phrase would be "a few endangered animals").

   some of these — quantifying adjective (some) and pronominal (these), referring back to some part of the group of "endangered animals" in line 1.

   others — pronominal, referring to some part of the group of "endangered animals" in line 1 and contrasting with the "some of these" in line 2.

   as — conjunction, indicating relationship both causal and temporal

   the animals' — word repetition, referring back to "endangered animals" in line 1.

   still other animals — "still other" is a quantifying adjective referring back to some part of the group of "endangered animals" in line 1, and contrasting with the "some of these" in line 2 and "others" in line 3. The child will need help understanding that the passage is discussing one group of animals, mentioned in line 1, which is divided into 3 parts, with the parts indicated by "some of these" in line 2, "others" in line 3 and "still other animals" in line 5.

2. **some disappear** — quantifying adjective, referring to a part of the group of animals mentioned in line 1, together with repetition of the word "disappear."

   other animals die — "other" is a contrasting adjective, referring to some part of the group of animals mentioned in line 1, and contrasting with the "some" in line 2, together with substitution of the word "die" as a synonym for "disappear."

   they — pronoun, referring the the word "animals" at the beginning of the sentence. Some children may need to be reminded that the antecedent for the pronoun is within rather than outside the same sentence.

   as — conjunction, indicating relationship both causal and temporal.

   when — conjunction, indicating temporal relationship.

   animals — word repetition, referring back to "animals" in line 1.

   also – adverb, conveying relationship of "in addition to," tying together pollution and lost habitats as causes of animal deaths.

   animal deaths — word substitution, referring back to "disappearing" in line 1 and "die" in line 2.

We have probably gone into much more detail here than you will need to go with any individual child. What we have tried to do is give an indication of the degree of cohesion present in even a brief, seemingly simple passage, any or all of which may be opaque to a child who is unaware of the importance of these devices. All of these are points to probe for comprehension on the child's part. It will probably not be necessary to label the nature of the cohesive device for the child, as we have done. This is a level of metalinguistic awareness unnecessary for a child's ability to comprehend cohesion. The key here is to find out which cohesive devices are causing difficulty for the child, by checking for comprehension, and then to help the child recognize and interpret the devices in text.

Taking the activity apart

Karen French, Melanie's clinician, asked the reading specialist in the school to give her some insight into Melanie's problems with reading comprehension. The teacher reported to her that Melanie seemed to have difficulty understanding how the information presented in paragraphs was related. She said, "She seems to see every sentence as an isolated fact, and she isn't able to understand how they relate to each other or to the main idea of the paragraph. That's why she has so much difficulty with reading comprehension, even though she can usually decode the words." As we reported at the end of Chapter 7, Karen had checked Melanie's comprehension of cohesive devices using the approach described in Appendix 3, so she was not surprised to hear what the reading specialist told her. Karen also discussed Melanie's difficulties with her classroom teacher, and they decided that after pre-teaching Melanie some cohesion identification strategies, Karen and the teacher would do a series of similar lessons with the entire class. Since Melanie will have already worked through and practiced the process, she should be able to do well in the classroom lessons.

As we discuss teaching the language impaired school age child the strategies needed for school success, we are dealing with concepts such as main idea, cohesion, inference, etc. as if each was a separate entity. In reality, they are all interrelated. Knowledge of cohesion helps identify the main idea by allowing a child to trace patterns of reference. However, it is sometimes difficult to spot cohesion without knowing the main idea of the text. The speech-language pathologist must understand and appreciate the interweaving of these concepts in order to recognize where the child's breakdown is occurring and in order to put the system back together after taking it apart to teach one concept at a time.

The first step in working with Melanie involved mediating—explaining to her what the focus of the activity would be, and why it was important. Karen French knew that she would need to work on a very concrete level. She took the text passage from Melanie's third grade Social Studies book quoted above, and typed it into the computer, printing it sentence by sentence, cutting the sentences apart, and gluing them on index cards. She began her session with the cards placed in the proper sequence on a large sheet of paper. She also had the page of the textbook open on the table in front of herself and Melanie. She said to Melanie:

Remember when your teacher explained to you about paragraphs and sentences? Paragraphs are all indented like this, aren't they? And every time we see indenting, we know we have a new paragraph. Every paragraph has several sentences in it. Remember that a sentence starts with a capital letter and ends with a period or question mark? Let's count the number of sentences in this paragraph. [They did this together.] Now, the sentences in a paragraph are usually all about the same thing, and they are all tied together in special kinds of ways. When we talk about how sentences are tied together, we're talking about cohesion. That's what we're going to start learning about today. Cohesion. It means tying sentences together in special ways. It's important to learn about cohesion, because if you understand cohesion, you will understand paragraphs in your textbooks much better. I have typed out this paragraph here on cards, so we can figure out cohesion without making marks in the book. We can do anything we want to with our cards, though. I've brought some highlighters here so we can make marks on them, and we can even move them around if we want to. First, let's read the paragraph and decide what it's about.

Karen read the paragraph aloud to Melanie, and then asked Melanie to read it to her. After they read it, they discussed what it might be about, and Karen gave Melanie her first strategy: **You can usually tell from the first sentence what a paragraph is about**. Karen had hesitated about teaching this strategy, because the topic of the paragraph is not always in the first sentence. However, after looking at Melanie's third grade textbooks, she decided there were very few exceptions to this, and that it would be easier to deal with exceptions once Melanie had some strategy for beginning her analysis. She asked Melanie to highlight the words in the first sentence that told what the paragraph was about. Melanie began by marking "animals," and they discussed why "endangered animals" might be a better choice, because it was more specific. Karen then asked Melanie to go through the paragraph and highlight every occurrence of the word "animals." She gave Melanie her second strategy: **We can tie sentences together by repeating the same key words over and over**. Melanie was surprised to notice how many times the word "animals" appeared in the paragraph. Then Karen said to her, *There are some other words in this paragraph that are substituting for "animals." Can you find any of them?* Melanie stalled here, and Karen decided to back up and work by analogy with personal pronouns, which she knew Melanie could comprehend. She wrote a three sentence paragraph as follows: *Melanie is a girl in third grade. Melanie likes to play jump rope at recess. Melanie likes pizza for lunch.* She reminded Melanie that they didn't have to keep saying "Melanie" over and over, and asked what word they might use instead. Melanie suggested "she," and Karen reminded her that a word that could take the place of a noun was called a pronoun. They listed several pronouns, such as "she," "he," "it," and "them." Karen then said, *sometimes we just substitute another noun. For example, we could say "the girl" instead of Melanie. Let's try to find some places in our paragraph where some other word has been used instead of "animals."* She took the card with the second sentence on it, and asked Melanie which word or words might tie this sentence back to "endangered animals" in the first sentence. Melanie pointed to the specific animals named, and they agreed that these words were good pointers. She gave Melanie her third strategy: **We can tie sentences together by substituting words that mean the same thing as the key words**.

Then Karen drew her attention to "few," and asked if Melanie knew what it meant. Melanie knew it meant "not very many," and Karen asked her if she thought they might put the phrase "endangered animals" after the word "few." They decided this would work, and Melanie pointed out that "few" was standing in for the phrase "few endangered animals." They decided to apply this strategy to the fourth sentence in the paragraph. Karen took the card and asked Melanie to find a word that was substituting for "animals." Tentatively, Melanie guessed "others," and was delighted to be able to highlight it.

Then Karen called Melanie's attention to the series of words "some," "others," and "still other." She pointed out to Melanie that these words often signalled a list, and that they would need to decide what was being listed. She took out one of her pre-drawn pies, a visual aid she used often in working with children like Melanie. She pointed out that the whole pie stood for the subject of the list, and each piece of the pie was one part of the whole. She said,

> *Let's let the whole pie be "endangered animals." That's what this paragraph is about, and that's what our list is about too. Now, what does the paragraph tell us about the pieces of the pie? I'll find the first piece. It is here, on this card that says "Some of these animals have become endan-*

gered because of too much hunting." So, I'll write "too much hunting" on this piece of the pie. Now, can you find another piece? Remember to look for our list words.

Melanie found the word "others" in the next sentence, and Karen asked her what the sentence said about this piece of the pie. They wrote "land development" on Melanie's piece. Then Karen encouraged Melanie to find the next list word. She located the phrase "still other," and they wrote "air and water pollution" on the next pie piece. When they had finished, the pie looked like the one shown in Figure 8–1.

Karen gave Melanie her final strategy: **Look for a list, and decide what is being listed.**

Putting the activity back together

Karen then went back over the four strategies, writing them down in a small notebook, which she kept for Melanie in her office, and also writing them on a card for Melanie to take away with her. They went back over the paragraph, and Melanie told Karen which strategy was being used in each sentence. Karen then gave Melanie the highlighter, and asked her to decide what the next paragraph in the text (photo-

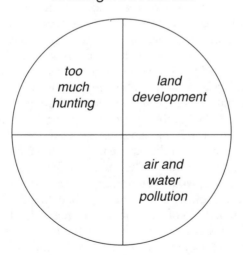

Endangered Animals

| too much hunting | land development |
| air and water pollution |

Figure 8–1. A visual organizer for paragraph cohesion.

copied by Karen for this purpose) was about, and then to highlight the cohesion words using her strategies. She reminded Melanie to read the whole paragraph before going back to the first sentence to try to decide what the paragraph was about. We have reprinted the paragraph below:

> Today, Americans as well as people around the world are trying to protect these animals and help them survive. Hunting laws are being changed. Land is being set aside for the animals to live on. Pollution is being controlled. Some zoos are even trying to raise endangered animals. But there is still much to be done. It is the duty of all people to show that they care for the earth and all the living things on it. (Joyce & Erickson, 1991, p. 277)

This paragraph was a difficult one for Melanie, because the key words in the first sentence were verbs ("protect" and "help"). Karen reminded Melanie to look for words that related to protecting and helping the animals. They agreed that it might be easier if they looked for phrases rather than single words, and Karen pointed out that "hunting laws changed" was one way to protect animals. She discovered that Melanie was not sure what it meant to "set aside" land, but once they had defined this concept, Melanie was able to find the cohesion words and phrases herself. Karen asked Melanie whether this paragraph had a list, and Melanie tried first to look for words like "other" and "some." When she didn't see these, she said there must not be a list. Karen took out another pie picture, and said, "OK, what did we agree that this paragraph might be about? Ways to protect and help animals. Let's write that over the pie, and see whether we can label the pieces of the pie." Once Melanie had the pie in front of her, she was able to look at the highlighted words in the paragraph and label the pieces. Karen then underlined the phrase "these animals" in the first sentence, and asked Melanie if she knew which animals the phrase was talking about. When Melanie hesitated, she took out a photocopied copy of the page of text on which both paragraphs appeared, and said, "Sometimes you have to look at the paragraph before the one you're reading. " Melanie was able to say that it must be talking about endangered animals, and Karen agreed. She drew a line from the phrase in paragraph 2 up to the phrase in paragraph 1 being referred to. The she asked Melanie if she saw any other ties between the two paragraphs. She suggested that Melanie use her strategies, and look at the words she had highlighted. Melanie quickly saw the repetition of the words "hunting," "land," and "pollution." This enabled Karen to point out that the list in paragraph 2 was directly related to the list in paragraph 1. Melanie could see this by looking at the two pies they had constructed.

Karen encouraged Melanie to apply her strategies whenever she read lessons in her textbook. She photocopied Melanie's Social Studies lessons for the next few weeks, so Melanie could use her highlighter to mark the cohesion words. She also gave Melanie several pie sheets, since the visualization seemed to be especially useful to her. She encouraged Melanie to bring the highlighted text and the pies to her sessions with Karen to discuss how she had applied her strategies.

A note about this activity

This is a highly metalinguistic activity. It demands that the child have the ability to talk about language and to focus on specific kinds of words, pulling them out from the meaningful text. A child who lacks this degree of metalinguistic awareness will not be able to focus on text at this level, and training metalinguistic awareness must come before work on cohesion. A case presented later in this chapter will address this need.

The third grade text Karen was working with uses repetition and substitution as major cohesive devices. Higher level texts, or texts written by different authors, are likely to involve more linguistically sophisticated cohesive devices, including conjunctions and causal or temporal adverbs. The same sort of strategies approach can be applied to helping the child with these cohesive devices, but comprehending them will demand more advanced cognitive understandings and more sophisticated vocabulary than Melanie has. When working with conjunctions, in particular, once the child seems to understand the functions of the words and their meanings, it is often useful to present texts with the conjunctions omitted and ask the child to help fill in the blanks. This exercise helps to sensitize the child to the importance of these words in the text.

Taking the activity into the classroom

The week before the scheduled team-teaching, Melanie's teacher chose paragraphs from the children's social studies book. She specifically chose from units the students had already covered to eliminate background information concerns. The teacher put a couple of the paragraphs on overheads. The class followed along while the teacher read the paragraph. Then, working with the class as a whole, Karen mediated for the children, explaining cohesion to them in the same way she had previously explained it to Melanie. Since finding the main idea of a paragraph is very difficult for children in third grade, the classroom teacher did this for them. Then, using the first paragraph on the overhead the classroom teacher and Karen highlighted certain words and asked leading questions to get the children to see how sentences were tied together. Karen asked Melanie to share with the class the four rules she had learned about cohesion. Melanie read her rules from the cards that Karen had given her during their individual session. Karen wrote the rules on the board for all the children. After the class read the second paragraph in unison, the teacher asked the children (calling on Melanie frequently) to identify the cohesive words and phrases. As they went through the paragraph identifying cohesive devices, Karen placed each word or phrase under the strategy that allowed the children to find it. Now the classroom teacher divided the class into small groups. Each group was given a paragraph, a highlighter, a pencil, and four sheets of paper with a strategy written at the top of each. Each paragraph already had the main idea highlighted. The children were told that as a group they should highlight the words or phrases that "tie the sentences together" and then write the word/phrase under the appropriate strategy. When the groups were finished, one person from each group was asked to read the paragraph and then another person from the group was asked to list what words/phrases they listed under which strategy. The classroom teacher liked the way this session went, so she decided to repeat the lesson on her own using other types of texts and in fact using the children's own writing to demonstrate how and when they might use cohesive devices. She was pleased to note that the children were getting better at comprehending cohesive devices in text, but disappointed that some of them, including Melanie, were still not using cohesive devices very well in their own texts. She met with Karen to discuss what might be done.

As she tried to think how to help Melanie and her classmates learn some strategies to turn this set of unconnected sentences into a paragraph, Karen reviewed the information about how children develop in their use of cohesive devices. As Irwin (1988) points out, children's ability to use the various cohesive devices develops throughout the elementary grades. Second graders use more personal pronouns than first graders. Between grades two and five, children shift from the use of one-word conjunctions to the inclusion of more complex syntax. While second graders tend to write generally unconnected, list-like prose, fourth graders can begin to connect to a main idea, and sixth graders mark connections not only to the main idea but also between sentences. Strategies to help children improve cohesion generally involve sentence and clause combining, replacing nouns with pronouns, and inserting conjunctions. Karen suggested that they begin with some of the children's oral narratives, knowing that the children who were struggling with cohesion were also the ones who hated to write. She suggested that if they could write down a few oral narratives, the children could work out ways to make them more cohesive. So, they began by choosing four children, including Melanie, to go to the back of the room to tell Karen about a videotape they had see about spiders. Karen began by asking the

children what they had liked best about the video. She got the following descriptions, one from each child:

*1. I liked the part about the trapdoor spiders. You know, they have this
nest in the ground and they have this little door, and whenever they
hear a bug coming along the ground they reach out and grab it, and the
bug never even sees the spider.*
*2. I liked how some spiders have these webs underground, in these kind
of tunnels, and they lie on their backs and a bug falls into the tunnel
and they just kind of curl their legs around it and eat it.*
*3. I liked the part about how spiders crawl up like on a tree stump or
some high place and they shoot a piece of spider web up and they can
grab it and fly through the air, like the baby spiders did at the end of
Charlotte's Web.*
*4. I liked all the pictures of spider webs, like these gigantic webs that
look like they have writing on them, and how spider webs are as strong
as steel, and how spiders wrap flies and stuff up in their webs and eat
them later on.*

At the beginning of the lesson for the class, Karen reminded them
that they had learned to recognize many cohesive devices in their textbooks. She pointed out to them that they used cohesion themselves
when they talked and wrote, but that they could all probably do a better job. She said, "There are some strategies we can all use when we
write to help make our writing more cohesive. I'll put these on the
board for you." She wrote:

1. Make sure you have a main idea.
2. Try to find a way to tie each sentence to the main idea by using
   a. pronouns
   b. repetition of key words
   c. substitutions
   d. lists

She reminded them that the four ways to tie sentences to the main
idea were the four kinds of cohesive ties they had learned to recognize
in other people's writing. Before coming into the room, Karen had typed
the children's oral narratives about spiders into the computer, eliminat-
ing all cohesive ties. Account #3 was as follows:

*Spiders crawl up on a tree stump or some high place. Spiders shoot a
piece of spider web up. Spiders can grab a piece of spider web. Spiders
can fly through the air. The baby spiders flew through the air at the end
of Charlotte's Web.*

The child who had given the original oral narrative was grouped
with four other children, and they were asked to turn this into a cohesive narrative, using the strategies Karen had written on the board. The

group decided that "Spiders can fly through the air" was the main idea, and their revised narrative was:

> *Spiders can fly through the air. They crawl up a tree stump or some high place. They shoot a piece of spider web up, and they can grab it and fly. The baby spiders flew through the air at the end of* Charlotte's Web.

Karen and the teacher were both pleased with the results of this episode, and Karen resolved to use it with Melanie as preteaching device when Melanie had writing assignments for class.

WORKING ON MAIN IDEA IDENTIFICATION

While working with Melanie on cohesion, Karen confirmed the classroom teacher's observation that Melanie had a great deal of difficulty deciding what a unit of text was about. The classroom teacher explained that Melanie's failure to do this would cause difficulty for Melanie in every academic area, including math. Since their co-teaching activity with cohesion had worked so well, Karen and the teacher decided to take the same approach with main idea. Karen first asked the teacher what vocabulary she wanted to use for this concept, since there are a variety of words and phrases to choose from, including "topic sentence," "important idea," "theme," etc. The teacher preferred to use "main idea," so they decided to stick with that label. Karen then gave the teacher a copy of James Baumann's chapter entitled "The Direct Instruction of Main Idea Comprehension Ability" (1986), and explained that she planned to use Baumann's approach when working with Melanie.

The goals and objectives Karen established for Melanie were as follows:

> **Goal:** Melanie will identify and summarize the main idea and supporting details of paragraphs in order to increase her comprehension of text.
> **Objectives:**
> Given a list of three, four, or five related words, Melanie will generate a main idea for the list.
> Given a complex sentence, Melanie will identify and summarize the main idea by finding the topic of the sentence plus what is said about the topic.
> Given a paragraph of text in which the main idea is explicitly stated, Melanie will identify and summarize the main idea of the paragraph.
> Given the main idea for a paragraph of text, Melanie will summarize the relevant supporting details.

Activities for Teaching

Teaching main idea is not simple. It is a complex concept, involving many higher level language processes which cause difficulties for the language impaired child. Identifying main idea involves bringing to bear world knowledge, knowledge of narrative structure, knowledge of cohesion, problem solving skills, and metalinguistic awareness. It is not surprising that even children who are not language impaired have difficulty with this task. Baumann (1986) presents a tentative developmental hierarchy of main idea tasks and relations. He cautions the potential user of the hierarchy that it is "based upon the best estimates from the research literature and from intuition and feedback from experienced classroom teachers" (p. 144). He gives approximate grade levels representing the lowest grade at which a particular task should be taught. Based on his sequence, as a beginning third grader, Melanie would be expected to find the main idea in lists of words, and also to summarize the main idea of a sentence by finding the topic plus what is said about the topic. In third grade, she would be expected to begin to identify and summarize main ideas and details explicitly and implicitly stated in paragraphs. Baumann's entire sequence is summarized in Table 8–1.

Bauman (1986) discusses a five step program for teaching main idea. The steps, including the activities Karen used with Melanie, are summarized below.

Step 1. Introduction

The student is provided with a purpose for the lesson. This is the step in which mediation must occur. Karen explained to Melanie that everything she reads whether it is a story or Science or Social Studies, has a main idea and many details that tell more about the main idea. Karen then went on to explain that when Melanie could find the main idea and state it in her own words her reading would improve and be more fun. She also explained that finding the main idea would help her remember what she read. Karen pointed out to Melanie that finding the main idea is really nothing more than a categorizing task similar to ones they had worked on before. She then moved on to Step 2.

Step 2. Example

Karen followed her mediation with an example to help Melanie understand the concept of main idea. She showed Melanie the following simple paragraph, typed in large type on a page:

TABLE 8–1. Sequence of main idea tasks.*

Task	Grade
Main ideas in lists of words	1 and up
Main ideas in sentences	2 and up
Main ideas and details in paragraphs where the main idea is explicitly stated	3 and up
Main ideas and details in paragraphs where the main idea is implicitly stated	3 and up
Main ideas and details in short passages where the main idea is explicit	5 and up
Main ideas and details in short passages where the main idea is implicit	5 and up
Main idea outlines for short passages where the main idea is explicit	6 and up
Main idea outlines for short passages where the main idea is implicit	6 and up
Main ideas in long passages (such as entire chapters in a textbook)	7 and up

*Based on Baumann (1986), pp. 145–147.

Farm animals are important to us. We get bacon from pigs. Our milk comes from cows. Chickens give us eggs.

Karen read the paragraph with Melanie and demonstrated how she identified the main idea and the details. She then moved to the next step in the instructional process.

Step 3. Direct instruction

In this step the clinician is leading the lesson by providing modeling to demonstrate the target behavior. The student should be actively involved in working with the text. To emphasize the categorization aspect of main idea, Karen prepared several word lists, each of which consisted of exemplars from a group, such as apples, pears, peaches, and asked Melanie to tell her how the words in each set were alike. As Karen expected, Melanie was able to do this easily. Karen explained to Melanie that she was actually finding the main idea for the list when she talked about how the words were alike. Referring to the list given above, she said "Fruit is the main idea of this list and the types of fruit listed are the supporting details." Karen and Melanie worked on several lists, some of which contained the main idea within the list (ie: baseball, hopscotch, tag, games, hide-and-seek). In this instruction step, Karen was teaching Melanie that sometimes the main idea is explicitly stated and sometimes it is implicit and that she could identify it either way.

Step 4. Teacher directed application

In this step the students are forced to apply the skill taught previously. The clinician is initiating the activity and is there for support and assistance if needed but the child bears more responsibility. Karen now provided Melanie with a list of words taken from the second grade Social Studies book. She moved back to the second grade book to be sure that Melanie was familiar with the concepts. Some of the lists contained the main idea and some did not. Melanie was required to state the main idea of each list. During this step, Karen observed carefully to determine whether Melanie needed further assistance. She had decided that if Melanie had any difficulty, she would introduce her to the umbrella visualization. This visualization uses a drawing of an umbrella, like the one shown in Figure 8-2. The main idea is written on the umbrella, and supporting details are written underneath. This helps the student remember that the main idea "covers" all the details.

Step 5. Independent practice

In this step Karen provided Melanie with materials that had not been used in previous instructions and asked her to complete them independently. Karen chose the words from the Social Studies unit that Melanie's class had just finished. She asked Melanie to do two tasks. One was to identify the main idea from a list of words and the other was to generate details for a main idea that Karen provided. For example, Karen gave the main idea "things we do at school," and Melanie provided details such as "reading," "math," and "recess."

Karen then followed steps three through five to help Melanie find and summarize the main idea and supporting details in complex sentences such as "Melanie, the girl with red hair, is in third grade." Although Melanie had learned to work with the word lists very quickly, she had a little more trouble with complex sentences. Karen realized

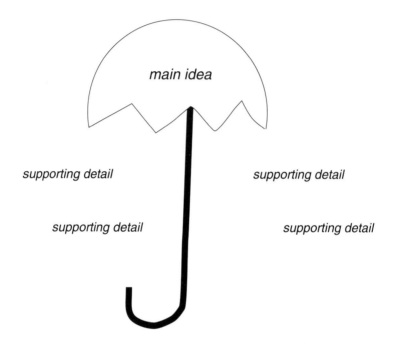

Figure 8–2. The main idea umbrella.

that her difficulties were in part related to her problems with metalinguistic awareness at the sentence level, and she made sure that the sentences she used all dealt with ideas Melanie was familiar with, and used vocabulary Melanie already knew, to reduce the processing demands of the task.

In their weekly planning meetings, Karen and Melanie's teacher decided that as Karen completed each teaching unit (lists of words, and main idea in a sentence) they would do a similar unit with the entire class. For the first lesson they designed the "Main Idea Game." The class was divided into groups of five children each, and each group was given a set of 12 cards containing words or short phrases. Karen and the teacher had made sure in advance that each set of cards contained one card that was clearly a main idea under which six of the cards could be grouped. The remaining cards contained unrelated words or phrases. For example one card set contained the following: *cat, dog, hamster, pets, elephant, pony, hippopotamus, dinosaur, guinea pig, rabbit, zebra, crocodile.* The children were asked to go through their cards, find the card they believed contained the main idea, and group with it the cards that contained the supporting details. When the groups had finished, each group was asked to tell the class about their sets, and explain why they had left some of their cards out. The teacher then asked each group of children whether they could put together the cards they had left out, and find a main idea for that set. The children who had the set listed above eventually put all the remaining cards except the "dinosaur" one into a set and called it "wild animals." They had an argument about whether dinosaurs should be included, since they were extinct. The teacher agreed with their decision not to include this card, and explained that if they called their main idea "wild animals living today," they would have a good reason to leave out dinosaurs. When the children had settled on their card sets and main ideas, each group was asked to put their main idea on an umbrella, and write a sentence related to the main idea for each supporting idea. The group mentioned above had as its main idea: *Many wild animals are alive today.* Their supporting ideas were: *Elephants are large animals and live in Africa. Crocodiles live in rivers in Africa. Zebras live on the plains of Africa and look like black and white horses. A hippopotamus might live in Africa or in the zoo.*

During the classroom activity, Karen functioned as coach for Melanie's group, helping them to think through the process for deciding which cards to include in their set and what the main idea for the set was. When Melanie's group was ready to write the paragraph, Karen sat with her to provide assistance. She helped her to compose a sentence about the word she was given, and helped her think through whether her word was a main idea or a supporting detail. She also helped the group think about how to make their sentences relate to the main idea, including Melanie in the discussion by asking her to suggest a word that might tie two of their sentences together.

Later in the semester Melanie's teacher asked Karen to join her in preparing instruction on identifying and summarizing the main idea from a paragraph. The teacher said that in a week the class would begin Chapter 4, "Using Resources in Rural Communities," in their Social Studies text. Karen and the teacher discussed how to use trade books to supplement the text and how to strengthen the children's skill with main idea. The teacher reported that many children in the class had trouble summarizing the main idea. She said they could find the sentence (it's usually the first sentence in the paragraph), but when they were asked what the main idea was, they simply read the first sentence. She was not sure they really understand and could put it in "their own words."

The teacher began the lesson by telling the children that the "topic/theme" of their new lesson would be farming. She asked them to think of as many words about farms and farming as they could. While they were brainstorming, Karen and the teacher wrote the words/phrases on the board as the children called them out. The teacher and Karen did not make any verbal or nonverbal comments during this exercise and accepted all responses whether related to the subject or not. (Since Melanie's teacher incorporated brainstorming into many of the class activities, the children were familiar with the rules of brainstorming). The teacher then presented and read the trade book about farming, *Heartland* by Diane Siebert. The purpose of the trade book at this point in the lesson is to stimulate the children's thinking, and help them to begin to call up what they already know about farms and farming. The children were encouraged to add to the brainstorming list anything they thought of during the reading of the trade book. Still using the trade book for support, the class was asked to generate some main ideas from the list on the board and from the book, and then group the words under the appropriate main idea. As they did this, Karen began to construct a series of "main idea webs" on the board, like those shown in Figure 8–3.

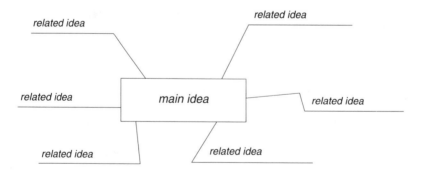

Figure 8–3. Main idea web.

Each child was then asked to look at the main idea and supporting details in one of the webs, and write a summary statement of the main idea. Since the main ideas were generated by the children in the first place and were not presented in sentence form the children were not able to use someone else's statement of the main idea, but had to generate their own summary statements. During this exercise, Karen and the teacher moved around the classroom, giving assistance. Karen spent most of her time with Melanie, making sure she understood the task and coaching as Melanie worked out a summary statement for one of the webs.

The children were then asked to read part A of Lesson 1 of the unit. After each child had read the section, the children were paired and each pair was asked to decide what the main idea of each paragraph was and to summarize it in writing in their own words. Karen acted as coach for Melanie and her partner. The teacher then called on two or three pairs to read the summary statements they had written, and the class as a whole decided whether they agreed. For part B of Lesson 1, each pair of children was provided with a worksheet using the umbrella or web visualization, and was asked to fill in the diagram with the main idea and the supporting details. Again, Karen acted as coach for Melanie and her partner.

Some Notes About These Activities

Working with main idea provides an opportunity to do pre-teaching with language impaired children. The purpose of pre-teaching is to give the language impaired child a head start. Since these children will generally need much more repetition and practice on complex language concepts like main idea, and since the classroom is not set up to allow for this redundancy, language intervention is a fine place to provide it. Pre-teaching will make it possible for the language impaired child to participate successfully in the classroom when the new concept is introduced. It is also important for the collaborating speech-language pathologist to be in the classroom to coach when possible. Karen's coaching helped Melanie remember what she had learned in the pre-teaching lessons, and helped her apply it to what was happening in class.

WORKING ON INFERENCING AND PREDICTING

Are inferencing and predicting parts of the same process? How are these related to "drawing conclusions?" In what order do we focus on these processes when teaching language impaired children? When we first asked outselves these questions it seemed as though they should be easy to answer. But the more we tried to separate these concepts from one another and from cohesion and main idea, the more confusing the issue became. It helped us to consider all of these concepts as being related to "critical thinking." It became clear to us that making predictions and drawing conclusions were based on the ability to infer meaning. In other words, to hypothesize a reasonable outcome, you need to use your past experiences and knowledge as well as the facts from the text or lecture to make an inference. In teaching language impaired students about inferencing, our goal should be to help them organize their ideas so they can access both "new" and "old" information when they need to make inferences.

Karen kept these ideas in mind as she established the following goal and objectives for Melanie:

> **Goal:** Melanie will develop strategies for inferencing to increase comprehension and literal memory for text.
> **Objective:** Melanie will establish logical categories for personal experiences.
> **Objective:** Melanie will indicate when her personal experiences are limited in a given area of study.
> **Objective:** Melanie will respond to cues to recall relevant personal experiences within the context of a shared book experience.
> **Objective:** Melanie will relate logical associations between her world knowledge ("old information") and information presented in text ("new information"), using visualization strategies.

Activities for Teaching

Taking the activity apart

The first step in teaching Melanie to make inferences involved explaining what inferencing was all about. Karen asked Melanie to tell what she knew about questions. Since Karen and Melanie had worked on formulating and responding to simple question in previous years, Karen was eager to see what Melanie's perceptions were at this stage of her development. Melanie described questions by saying, "Some are easy, some are hard." Karen then reviewed the definition of a question taught to Melanie by her second grade teacher. Karen said, "Remember, a question is a sentence that asks you something." Karen and Melanie practiced asking one another simple questions. Then they wrote their definition of a question in Melanie's Social Studies log. (The Social Studies log was a spiral notebook in which Melanie kept her vocabulary words, notes, and answers to review questions.) Next, Karen asked Melanie how she figured out the answers to questions that her teacher asked during class discussion. Melanie explained that she "just knew" the easy ones, and "couldn't do" the hard ones. Then Karen asked her how she answered the questions from the textbook. Melanie explained that sometimes she looked at the pictures, and sometimes her dad helped her.

Karen concluded that Melanie's understanding of the process of finding answers to questions related to her texts did not seem to involve reflecting on what she knew, thinking about what additional information she might need, or where to find it. Karen explained to Melanie that sometimes the questions she thought were hard required her to "make inferences." She explained:

> When you use information you already have to understand something new, you are making an inference.

Together, they wrote this sentence in Melanie's social studies log. Karen decided to try a short exercise, to see whether Melanie had understood the idea. She said:

> I am going to describe my friend John to you, and when I've finished, I want you to tell me what job you think John has. Ready? John gets up early every morning and goes to the barn to milk the cows. Then he feeds the chickens and the hogs. After breakfast, he gets on his tractor and drives out to the field. Yesterday he planted his new corn crop. What is John's job?

Karen knew that Melanie lived on a farm, and that her own father did many of the tasks she had described. Melanie was able to answer that John was a farmer. Then Karen said, "How did you know that, Melanie?" Melanie looked confused, and replied, "I just did." Karen explained to Melanie that she knew what John's job was because she knew a lot about farmers, and she was able to use what she already knew to answer the new question. They then tried another example, which Karen chose because Melanie said she wanted to be a veterinarian when she grew up. Karen said:

> My friend Andrea goes to her office every morning. She puts on a white coat. All day long she sees sick animals. Sometimes she gives them a shot to make them feel better. What is Andrea's job?

Of course, Melanie knew at once that Andrea was a vet. Karen said, "What did you know about veterinarians that helped you answer that question?" Melanie replied that she knew that they helped sick animals. Karen then asked, "How did you know that?" Melanie explained that she had taken her kitten to the vet when it was sick, and the vet had showed her the scales she used to weigh animals, and had let her hold the kitten while he gave it a pill. Karen pointed out, "You knew about veterinarians because you had some personal experience with them, didn't you? Well, that's how we know a lot of things. And when we are asked a question, sometimes we need to think about our personal experience to decide whether we know about the answer to the question." Let's try another example.

> I'm going to tell you about what's happening, and you tell me what time of day it is. Ready? The children all lined up at the door of the classroom. The walked down the hall in a line, and went into the cafeteria. Each child picked up a tray and walked down the food line to decide what to eat. Now, before you answer my question, tell me, have you ever done this?

Melanie nodded her head.

And what time of day was it when you did it?

Melanie replied that it was lunchtime, or 12:00. Again, Karen pointed out to Melanie that she had used her own experience to help her answer the question. She then continued:

> What you have been doing is making inferences, Melanie. That is something we all do when we read. We understand a lot about what we are reading because we have had experiences that help us to know what the text means. If you will use your inferencing ability, you'll have a much easier time with some of the hard questions in social studies. And what will happen if you can answer more of the hard questions?

Melanie thought for a minute, and said that she would get better grades on her tests. Karen agreed, and said, "Now you know why inferencing is important. It will help you get better grades. And if you want to go to school to become a vet, it's important for you to get good grades."

An Activity Outside the Classroom

Karen decided to begin by giving Melanie a set of strategies she could use to remind her about inferencing, no matter which school subject she was working with. She particularly wanted Melanie to be able to deal with the questions at the ends of the chapters in her science and social studies books. She gave Melanie a sheet of paper with the following three strategies printed on it:

STRATEGY # 1: READ THE QUESTION AND CHANGE IT INTO A FILL-IN-THE-BLANK SENTENCE. UNDERLINE THE IMPORTANT WORDS. THEN ASK YOURSELF, "WHAT IS THIS ABOUT?"

STRATEGY #2: WRITE DOWN WHAT YOU KNOW ABOUT THE MAIN IDEA OF THE QUESTION. USE YOUR PERSONAL EXPERIENCES (WHAT YOU HAVE SEEN, READ, OR HEARD) TO GIVE YOU IDEAS.

STRATEGY #3: READ THE QUESTION AGAIN. MAKE A FEW INFERENCES BASED ON CONCRETE INFORMATION FROM THE TEXT AND YOUR LIST OF WHAT YOU KNOW.

With the strategies in front of them, Karen and Melanie then looked at a social studies lesson Melanie had already had, related to natural resources and how communities used them. Karen chose this lesson because many of the questions in the text itself called for inferences. For example, the reader was asked, "If you were planning a new community, would you cut down all the trees? Would you build houses or a community park near the river?" Karen asked Melanie to pretend that she was in charge of building a town. The land where the town would be built had trees, a river, two steep hills, and some flat land. She put on the table a piece of paper with these features drawn on it, as shown in Figure 8-4.

Then she gave Melanie some small wooden houses taken from a Monopoly set, together with some small pictures cut from magazines of a church, people playing in a park, a farmyard, and a corn field. She asked Melanie to help her decide where the people's houses, and the other parts of the town she had in front of her, should go. Melanie gave much thought to placing the features of the town, and then Karen referred her to the questions from the text. She said, "Would you cut down all the trees, Melanie?" Melanie immediately said no. Then Karen said,"OK, let's talk about that. Why would you keep the trees?" Melanie answered that they would give shade, and that they would be there for children to climb in. Karen agreed that these were good reasons for not cutting down all the trees, but that not everyone would like to have trees growing everywhere. Then Karen took the picture of the corn field, and said, "The farmer who wanted to plant this field, cut down the trees. Why did he do this? Let's use our strategies to figure that out." First, they rephrased the question as follows: The farmer cut down the trees because _____. Then they decided that the important words in the question were "farmer," and "cut down the trees." Then Karen asked Melanie to think about her father's farm, and tell her whether there were trees in the middle of the corn field. Melanie agreed that there were none. Karen said, "What do you think might happen if there

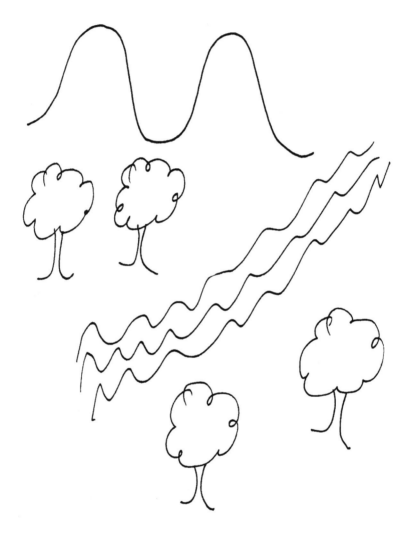

Figure 8–4. Melanie's community map.

were trees in the corn field?" Melanie couldn't answer the question, and Karen knew that she needed to help Melanie establish a better set for calling up her knowledge. As she frequently did, she turned to a trade book, in this case *Farming* by Gail Gibbons. As Karen and Melanie read the book together and looked at the pictures, Karen called Melanie's attention to all the pictures of the corn field. When they finished the book, Karen said, "Were there any trees in the corn field?" Melanie agreed that there had been none. Karen asked, "What did you see in the field?" Melanie looked back at the pictures and answered, "Tractor, combine." Karen pointed to Strategy 2 on Melanie's list. "So," she said, "what could we write down here? Let's write down that tractors and combines have to work in corn fields." Then Karen asked, "So what would happen if there were trees?" Melanie immediately replied, "The tractor and the combine would run into them." "Good. Now, read the question again. Why did the farmer cut down the trees?" Melanie answered quickly, "So the tractor and the combine wouldn't run into them." Karen then went back over the three strategies, helping Melanie to see what they had done at every point in the process, and reminding her again that she had answered the question based on information she got from her own experience, in this case, from reading a book about farming. Melanie needed several activities such as this one to learn to call up her background knowledge and apply it in new situations. Karen then called Melanie's attention back to the model town she had constructed, and referred her to the second question. "Would you put houses near the river, or would you put a community park near the river?" Melanie had put a park on one side of the river and houses on the other side. Karen asked her to talk about this layout. Melanie responded that some people could live near the river and catch fish for their food, and other people could go to the park so the children could play in the water and people could put their boats in the river. Karen said, "How did you know that people might want to play in the water, and put their boat in, and catch fish?" Melanie replied, "Because that's what we do on our river." Karen reminded her again that she had used her own knowledge to make inferences and answer questions in her textbook.

Taking the Activity Into the Classroom

Meanwhile, Melanie's teacher, knowing that Karen was working on inferencing with Melanie, asked Karen to come into the classroom to do some teaching, both for Melanie and for the rest of the class. Their Social Studies unit was on Farming in the United States, and the teacher pointed out that the first question at the end of the chapter called for inferencing by the students. It read, "In your opinion, why were many farms quite small long ago?" The answer to this question was not given anywhere in the chapter. The relevant textual passage was, "A farm set like this shows what many farms were like years ago, when a family could do most of the work with a few machines. There are still small farms like this in the United States. But today many farms are very large" (Joyce & Erickson, 1991, p. 73). Karen agreed to come into the classroom and teach the whole class the three strategies she had been helping Melanie to use. They went through the exercise of rephrasing the question, and identified "farms," "small," and "long ago" as the important words. Then Karen told the class that she was not an expert about farms, although she knew that many of them lived on farms. She suggested that, before they moved to Strategy 2, they should share some books she had brought in about farming. She divided the class into groups, and each group was given one of a group of books related to farms that the school librarian had helped Karen find. Each group was asked to read and look at their book, and when they had finished, to make a list of the ideas they had from the books and from their own knowledge about farms. Each group was given a large piece of paper on which to write their ideas. Karen worked with Melanie's group, and the teacher walked around the room from group to group, to help the children stay focused on the task and to answer questions. Melanie's group wrote down the following ideas:

farms grow food	farms have apples
farms have animals	farms have cows
farms have baby animals	farms get tornados
farmers use machines	farms need land
people work on farms	farms grow soybeans and corn

The groups were all asked to share the ideas they had written down. Then Karen pointed to Strategy 3, and asked the class whether they had any ideas about small farms. One student said, "My grandpa's farm used to be small a long time ago, but now it's big. He just got a new big gigantic tractor with air conditioning in it." The teacher asked why his grandpa had bought a new tractor, and the student replied that it made him able to get the work done much faster. The teacher then focused the class back on the question they were trying to answer, and asked "Can anyone use the information we now have about farms to say why some farms are big and some farms are small?" Karen suggested to Melanie and the others in her group that they look at the second page of their trade book, *Farming* by Gail Gibbons, which had pictures of a small farm and a big farm. She asked how they were different. Melanie raised her hand and said, "The big farm has machines to do the work." Karen coached, "And long ago, we didn't have so many . . . " "machines!" Melanie added. At that point, every hand in the class shot up with the answer to the fill-in-the-blank sentence. The teacher printed out the three strategies in large type on the computer, and posted them on the bulletin board in the classroom to help the students remember to use them when they encountered inferencing questions.

A Note About this Activity

As we always try to do, we have focused our activity around a set of strategies which can be appled to any subject matter the child might be working with. We have not addressed the issue of helping children to decide whether a question is answered in the text or whether it calls for inferencing. In the textbook Melanie's class was using, inferencing questions are always indicated by phrases such as "In your opinion," or "Why, do you think?" It would be important for many children to help them identify these conventions in their textbooks.

We have also chosen not to address individual types of inferences separately. This can be done, of course, if a child is having particular difficulty with a specific kind of inferencing, such as causal. In general, the strategies we teach children should suffice regardless of the kinds of inferences children are being asked to make. If a child is unable to employ the strategies, it is usually a sign that the activity is too high-level, and that preliminary work may need to be done on other aspects of text comprehension, such as cohesion and main idea, or even on vocabulary development.

SUMMARY

Text presents many language impaired children with the greatest challenge they will face in school. Many of them approach it with a mind set that says "I can't do this," either because they have had repeated experiences with failure in other language realms or because their first encounters with text resulted in failure. In general, children whose homes contain a great deal of print and who were read to as preschoolers will be less intimidated by their initial encounters with text. Unfortunately, many language impaired children do not come from these sorts of homes, and this puts an extra burden on speech-language pathologists and teachers who must provide these children with successful, interesting, entertaining encounters with the printed word. In spite of the fact that the activities in this chapter have focused on taking text apart, we feel that it is impossible to overemphasize the importance of making sure the child continues to interact with whole, meaningful texts, whether these are the school textbooks or trade books from the library.

CHAPTER 9

Putting the Book Aside

As you move from the pages of this book to the world of hands-on work with language impaired children, there are a few generalizations we want you to take with you. These relate to how we define ourselves and our work, how we accomplish change, and how we view language.

DEFINING OURSELVES

As we pointed out in Chapter 2, for too long speech-language pathologists in the schools have been content to be known as "speech teachers," working in small rooms set apart from everything else that happens in the school. The first step in self-definition for many professionals involves getting "language" into the label for what we do. Unless we educate those around us to the fact that we can and do work with children's language, we are not likely to get the sorts of referrals we need to help children. Many teachers and school speech-language pathologists are accustomed to thinking of language as a matter of words and sentences. They have difficulty conceiving of language processes that govern how we put sentences together to accomplish conversation and narrative. Because of this difficulty, children who need help are falling through the cracks. One speech-language pathologist of our acquaintance, recently hired to work on an assessment team for a large school system, told the horrifying story of finding a 12-year-old boy who had been held back in kindergarten at age 6 years, and still was able to read only at a second grade level. He had never had speech-language services, in spite of the fact that he was unable to retell a story with any complete episodes, or to make inferences. His phonological awareness was that of a 6 year old. Why had he never received services? Because the speech-language clinician in his school worked with articulation, fluency, and surface manifestation of morphological or syntactic problems such as past tense morphemes and pronoun confusions. Nobody in the school ever suggested that she should work with this child, because she had educated them about what she was and was not prepared to do. The moral of this story is that **we are the only people who can make sure we are seen as educators, who have an important contribution to make to children's academic success.** Defining ourselves in this way will demand that we see ourselves as continuing learners. We cannot expect to succeed if we base all our ideas on what we learned in school 10 or 15 years ago. New research is published every year. New ideas about intervention are presented in our journals and at state and national meetings. Continuing education will become a way of life for us, and we will profit as much as our clients.

Another part of seeing ourselves as educators involves perceiving the real value of collaboration. We must accept the fact that we are not the only people who can facilitate children's language development. We may be the ones who have the expertise and the relevant vocabulary to set goals and objectives, but we have an obligation to share that vocabulary and expertise at every opportunity. For the child's sake, we must not be seen as the only ones who can work with the child to meet goals. If that happens, the whole base for collaborating and working within the classroom will crumble. Everyone who works with a child, in whatever capacity, must come to feel ownership in that child's program. That includes parents, teachers, support personnel, and the child him or herself. There is no room for turf battles and jealous guarding of information in the education of children.

Just as we must come to recognize that other people in the child's life can facilitate language learning, we must also come to trust the instincts of those who refer children to us. Teachers don't pull children out of a hat to refer for speech-language assessment. If a teacher (or a parent, or a principal) requests an assessment, it is because there is some problem. It may not always be a speech or language problem, but we can't know this until we take an unbiased look at the child. The more we talk with other educators, the more we will learn about what they see when they interact with children, and the more they will learn about what we see. This was brought home to us recently when we had completed exhaustive language assessments of all the kindergartners in three local schools, for research purposes. We had told the kindergarten teachers what we were doing, but had not shared our results with them.

At the end of the year, we went back to each teacher with a list of the children in her class and the test results. As we sat down with one teacher, we said "There are only three children in your classroom we have concerns about." She responded, "I'll bet I can tell you who they are." And she named the three children we had identified as having problems with language. She said, "Of course, they don't have speech problems. But all three of them have struggled with phonics, and they just don't seem ready to do first grade work. I've recommended all three of them for transitional placement." When we explained the kinds of testing we had done, and what we had found, she pleaded with us to share the results with the first grade teachers, saying, "This is exactly the kind of thing we pay attention to in the classroom, but I had no idea there was actually a way to test kids for it." Essentially, we had managed to quantify the instincts of an experienced teacher, and in doing so, we gave her more confidence in her instincts and ourselves more confidence in our assessment approaches.

ACCOMPLISHING CHANGE

We realize that the kind of school practice we have described in this book will be both appealing and completely foreign to many professionals. A word of caution is in order: if you work in a more traditional practice, you must not expect to change to a collaborative, classroom based practice overnight. Change takes time. Not days and weeks of time, but sometimes years of time. Be patient. But don't stop. It is crucial for the future of school practice that we be willing to change. Educational reform is a reality. Schools are going to change. This is a time of transition, and as such, it is an ideal time for us to be proposing changes. If we aren't going to get left behind by the year 2000, we must embrace changes in service delivery. We must begin to work together to develop new models. This is our obligation, and, in our view, to refuse it is unethical. **Ask yourself: if not me—who? If not now—when?**

As you begin to move toward change, we hope you'll use this book as a resource, not as a cookbook. The activities we describe here are only examples of the sorts of things you can do with and for children. We don't have any magic insights into the one, true way. In fact, we aren't even sure there is a one, true way. See this book as a beginning, not as an end point. Get creative. Talk with other creative educators. Experienced teachers know what turns kids on. Get to know your school librarian and start reading children's books. Some of our best ideas have come from children's literature. Talk to parents about their children.

They know their own children, and they will also share with you their hopes and dreams for them—hopes and dreams you may be able to build on as you work with their children.

As you plan your intervention program, we believe it is important to let the child's Individual Educational Plan work for both the child and you. The goals and objectives you set down in the IEP must drive your practice with the child. Too often, we find that the IEP is regarded as a document that lives in the child's folder in the office rather than as a framework for action. One of the reasons we spelled out goals and objectives as we did in the book was to give some examples of how to write these for the aspects of language we chose to focus on. We also wanted to give you examples of how to turn goals and objectives into focused activities. Not only must the goals and objectives drive the intervention activities, they must also drive our attempts to demonstrate intervention efficacy. It is second nature for many clinicians to phrase objectives in terms of percentages of occurrence for specific language forms (for example, "Billy will use past tense -ed 85% of the time in obligatory contexts."). We have not put percentages in our objectives, in part because we can't come up with a good theoretical basis for doing it. But that doesn't mean that you can't count, if counting is important. When you observe a child as part of your initial assessment, note how often the child introduces an unmarked topic shift in a conversation. Note how many episodes the child can retell from a given story. Then look for quantitative evidence of change. There are some school environments which make this sort of demonstration absolutely essential. In other cases, the benefits of services may be viewed in the context of the IEP as a whole, and the child's improved academic performance or improved relationships with the peer group may be taken as evidence that the child is benefitting from services. Accountability is an important part of education reform, and the IEP should be viewed as the document that spells out what you will be held accountable for.

HOW WE VIEW LANGUAGE

It will be obvious to anyone who has read this book that we view language as something beyond words and sentences. Our focus has been on how children are able to use the words and syntax they know in the service of communication, both spoken and written, in the classroom and in the peer group. One linguistically oriented child language researcher of our acquaintance growls at us: "What you're talking about isn't language." Our response is, "It may not be what you think of as language, but language acquisition involves more than learning how to put words together to make sentences." For too many years, we have given lip service to the concept that language is a tri-partite phenomenon, consisting of content, form, and use. We work with content under the heading of cognitive development or sometimes lexical semantics. We work ad nauseam with form, under the heading of phonology, morphology, and syntax. But use gets left out in the cold. We think it's time to restore our view of language to equilibrium.

Obviously, defining language as we do affects our ability to use commercially available, standardized tests. In Chapter 1, we made a strong case against using such tests to determine who is language impaired. The main reason for this is that these tests are primarily focused on vocabulary, morphology, and syntax. They do not, for the most part, assess the higher level language processes underlying conversation, narrative, and reading and writing. Since these are precisely the processes school-aged language impaired children have problems with, using tests of morphology and syntax to try to identify school aged language impaired children is inappropriate. This does not mean that such tests should never be used with school-aged children. We have used them throughout this book, not to tell us who is language impaired, but rather to give us information about a child's language performance with vocabulary, morphology, and syntax. Test scores will never substitute for the information obtained from observing the child's language use in real contexts. If you can view a test as just another, rather specialized, context for finding out something about a child's language use, you will be approaching the perspective we have taken.

In the course of talking about language use in this book, we have taken the phenomenon apart. There's no other way to talk about it. In reality, though, "wholism" (to coin a term) is the only valid approach. To begin with, aspects of language use such as cohesion or metalinguistic awareness don't function in isolated contexts. We talked about metalinguistic awareness as we described intervention activities for conversation as well as when we discussed the child's problems with reading. We talked about cohesion in regard to text, but cohesion is also a part of maintaining topic in a conversation. Figuring out the topic of a conversation has much in common with figuring out the main idea of a paragraph. Script frameworks will support conversational participation as well as event recounting. It will be important for us to remember this as we begin to plan intervention activities. When we work with a particular aspect of language, we must go across contexts of use. In addition, it is unlikely that we will ever find a child who has problems with main idea comprehension and nothing else, or problems with topic maintenance and nothing else. Although we used our case studies as opportunities to focus in on a particular aspect of language, if we were working with these children in reality, we would need to work on several aspects. By keeping in mind the commonalities across contexts, we will find this easier to plan.

IN CONCLUSION

There always seems to be one last thing we need to say, one final admonition. We have four final admonitions for you:

Question.

Think.

Strive for the ideal

Welcome the challenges.

References

Ackerman, B. P. (1986). Referential and causal coherence in the story comprehension of children and adults. *Journal of Experimental Child Psychology, 41*, 336–366.

American Speech-Language-Hearing Association (1989, March). Issues in determining eligibility for language intervention. *ASHA*, 113–118.

Andersen, E. (1977). Young children's knowledge of role-related speech differences: A mommy is not a daddy is not a baby. *Papers and Reports on Child Language Development, 13*, 83–90.

Applebee, A. (1978). *The child's concept of story.* Chicago: University of Chicago Press.

Aram, D., Morris, R., & Hall, N. (1993). Clinical and research congruence in identifying children with specific language impairment. *Journal of Speech and Hearing Research, 36*, 580–591.

Ball, E., & Blachman, B. (1991). Does phoneme awareness training in kindergarten make a difference in early word recognition and developmental spelling? *Reading Research Quarterly, 26*, 49–66.

Bamberg, M. (1987). *The acquisition of narratives.* New York: Mouton de Gruyter.

Bashir, A. (1986). The continuum of language success and failure. Reaction discussion presented at the Language Learning Disabilities Institute, Boston, MA: Emerson College.

Bashir, A., Kuban, K., Kleinman, S., & Scavuzzo, S. (1983). Issues in language disorders: Considerations of cause, maintenance, and change. In J. Miller, D. Yoder, & R. Schiefelbush (Eds.) *ASHA Report No. 12* (pp. 92–106). Rockville, MD: American Speech-Language-Hearing Association.

Baumann, J. (1986). The direct instruction of main idea comprehension ability. In J. Baumann (Ed.), *Teaching main idea comprehension* (pp. 133–176). Newark, DE: International Reading Association.

Beaumont, C. (1992). Language intervention strategies for Hispanic LLD students. In H. Langdon & L. Cheng (Eds.). *Hispanic children and adults with communication disorders* (pp. 272–342). Gaithersburg, MD: Aspen.

Bennett-Kastor, T. (1983). Noun phrases and coherence in child narratives. *Journal of Child Language, 10*, 135–149.

Bishop, D. V. M., & Adams, C. (1992). Comprehension problems in children with specific language impairment: Literal and inferential meaning. *Journal of Speech and Hearing Research, 35*, 119–129.

Bishop, D. V. M., & Adams, C. (1991). What do referential communication tasks measure? A study of children with specific language impairment. *Applied Psycholinguistics, 12,* 199–215.

Bishop, D. V. M., & Adams, C. (1990). A prospective study of the relationship between specific language impairment, phonological disorders and reading retardation. *Journal of Child Psychology and Psychiatry, 31,* 1027–1050.

Bishop, D. V. M., & Adams, C. (1989). Conversational characteristics of children with semantic-pragmatic disorder. II: What features lead to a judgement of inappropriacy? *British Journal of Disorders of Communication, 24,* 241–263.

Bishop, D. V. M., & Rosenbloom, L. (1987). Classification of childhood language disorders. In W. Yule & M. Rutter (Eds.), *Language development and disorders* (Clinics in Developmental Medicine no. 101/102). London: MacKeith Press.

Blachman, B. (1991). Early intervention for children's reading problems: Clinical applications of the research in phonological awareness. *Topics in language disorders, 12,* 51–65.

Blachman, B. (1984). Language analysis skills and early reading acquisition. In G.P. Wallach & K.G. Butler (Eds.). *Language learning disabilities in school-age children* (pp. 271–287). Baltimore, MD: Williams & Wilkins.

Blachman, B., Ball, E., Black, S., & Tangel, D. (1991). Promising practices for beginning reading instruction: Teaching phoneme awareness in the kindergarten classroom. Manuscript submitted for publication.

Blank, M., & Marquis, A. (1987). *Teaching discourse.* Tucson, AZ: Communication Skill Builders.

Bower, G.H., Black, J.B., & Turner, T.J. (1979). Scripts in memory for text. *Cognitive Psychology, 11,* 177–220.

Bradley, L., & Bryant, P. (1985). *Rhyme and reason in reading and spelling.* International Academy for Research in Learning Disabilities Monograph Series, No. 1. Ann Arbor, MI: University of Michigan Press.

Bradley, L., & Bryant, P. (1983). Categorizing sounds and learning to read: A causal connection. *Nature, 30,* 419–421.

Brinton, B., & Fujiki, M. (1982). A comparison of request-response sequences in the discourse of normal and language-disordered children. *Journal of Speech and Hearing Disorders, 47,* 57–63.

Bruner, J. (1983). *Child's talk: Learning to use language.* Oxford: Oxford University Press.

Bryan, T., Donahue, M., & Pearl, R. (1981). Learning disabled children's communicative competence on referential communication tasks. *Journal of Pediatric Psychology, 6,* 383–393.

Catts, H. (1993). The relationship between speech-language impairments and reading disabilities. *Journal of Speech and Hearing Research, 36,* 938–958.

Catts, H. (1989). Phonological processing deficits and reading disabilities. In A. Kamhi & H. Catts (Eds.), *Reading disabilities: A developmental language perspective.* Boston: Allyn & Bacon.

Cazden, C. (1974). Play with language and metalinguistic awareness: One dimension of language experience. *The Urban Review, 7,* 28–39.

Craig, H., & Gallagher, T. (1986). Interactive play: The frequency of related verbal responses. *Journal of Speech and Hearing Research, 29,* 375–383.

Crais, E., & Chapman, R. (1987). Story recall and inferencing skills in language/learning disabled and nondisabled children. *Journal of Speech and Hearing Disorders, 52,* 50–55.

Damico, J. (1991). Clinical discourse analysis: A function approach to language assessment. In C. S. Simon (Ed.), *Communication Skills and Classroom Success* (pp. 125–149). Eau Claire, WI: Thinking Publications.

Dickenson, D. & McCabe, A. (1991). A social interactionist account of language and literacy development. In J. Kavanaugh (Ed.), *The language continuum* (pp.1–40). Parkton, MD: York Press.

Donahue, M., and Bryan, T. (1984). Communicative skills and peer relations of learning disabled adolescents. *Topics in Language Disorders, 4,* 10–21.

Elbow, G., & Greenfield, G. (1991). *Western hemisphere.* Morristown, NJ: Silver Burdett & Ginn.

Ellis Weismer, S. (1985). Constructive comprehension abilities exhibited by language-disordered children. *Journal of Speech and Hearing Research, 28,* 175–184.

Fazio, B., Naremore, R., & Connell, P. (1983). Tracking children at risk for specific language impairment. Paper presented to the American Speech-Language-Hearing Association, Anaheim, CA.

Feagans, L. (1982). The development and importance of narratives for school adaptation. In L. Feagans & D. Farran (Eds.), *The language of children reared in poverty* (pp. 95–116). New York: Academic Press.

Feagans, L., & Short, E. (1984). Developmental differences in the comprehension and production of narratives by reading disabled and normally achieving children. *Child Development, 55,* 1727–1736.

Feuerstein, R. (1979). *The dynamic assessment of retarded performers: The learning potential assessment device, theory, instruments, and techniques.* Baltimore: University Park Press.

Fey, M., & Leonard, L. (1983). Pragmatic skills of children with specific language impairment. In T. Gallagher and C. Prutting (Eds.), *Pragmatic assessment and intervention issues in language* (pp. 69–87). San Diego: College-Hill Press.

Fivush, R. (1984). Learning about school: The development of kindergartners' school scripts. *Child Development, 55,* 1697–1709.

Fivush, R., & Slackman, E. (1986). The acquisition and development of scripts. In K. Nelson (Ed.), *Event knowledge: Structure and function in development.* Hillsdale, NJ: Erlbaum.

Fowler, P. C. (1986). Cognitive differentiation of learning disabled children on the WISC-R: A canonical model of achievement correlates. *Child Study Journal, 16,* 25–37.

Fox, B., & Routh, D. (1975). Analyzing spoken language into words, syllables, and phonemes: A developmental study. *Journal of Psycholinguistic Research, 4,* 331–342.

Frederiksen, C.H. (1981). Inference in preschool children's conversations—a cognitive perspective. In J. Green & C. Wallat (Eds.), Ethnography and language in educational settings (pp.303–334). *Advances in Discourse Processes, Vol.V.* Norwood, N.J.: Ablex.

Gallagher, T., & Darnton, B. (1978). Conversational aspects of the speech of language disordered children: Revision behaviors. *Journal of Speech and Hearing Research, 21,* 118–135.

German, D. (1986). *Test of Word Finding.* Allen, TX: DLM Teaching Resources.

Gillam, R., & Johnston, J. (1992). Spoken and written language relationships in language/learning-impaired and normally achieving school-age children. *Journal of Speech and Hearing Research, 35,* 1303–1315.

Golinkoff, R. M. (1978). Critique: Phonemic awareness skills and reading achievement. In F. B. Murray & J. J. Pikulski (Eds.). *The acquisition of reading: Cognitive, linguistic and perceptual prerequisites.* Baltimore, MD: University Park Press.

Graybeal, C. (1981). Memory for stories in language impaired children. *Applied Psycholinguistics, 2,* 269–283.

Grice, H. P. (1975). Logic and conversation. In P. Cole, & J. Morgan (Eds.), *Syntax and semantics: Vol. 3. Speech acts.* New York: Academic Press.

Halliday, M. A. K. (1975). Development of texture in child language. In T. Myers (Ed.), *The development of conversation and discourse.* Edinburgh: Edinburgh University Press.

Halliday, M. A. K. & Hasan, R. (1976). *Cohesion in English.* London: Longman.

Hammill, D. (1991). *Detroit Test of Learning Aptitude-3.* Austin, TX: Pro-Ed.

Heath, S. (1986). Taking a cross-cultural look at narratives. *Topics in language disorders, 7,* 84–94.

Hresko, W., Reid, D., & Hammill, D. (1981). *The Test of Early Language Development.* Austin, TX: Pro-Ed.

Hudson, J., & Nelson, K. (1983). Effects of script structure on children's story recall. *Developmental Psychology, 19,* 625–635.

Irwin, J. (1988). Linguistic cohesion and the developing reader/writer. *Topics in Language Disorders, 8,* 14–23.

Johnson, D. D., & von Hoff Johnson, B. (1986). Highlighting vocabulary in inferential comprehension. *Journal of Reading, 29,* 622–625.

Joyce, W., & Erickson, R. (1991). *Comparing communities.* Morristown, NJ: Silver Burdett & Ginn.

Kamhi, A. (1987). Metalinguistic abilities in language impaired children. *Topics in Language Disorders, 7,* 1–12.

Kamhi, A., & Catts, H. (1986). Toward an understanding of developmental language and reading disorders. *Journal of Speech and Hearing Disorders, 51,* 337–347.

Kamhi, A., Catts, H., Koenig, L., & Lewis, B. (1984). Hypothesis-testing and nonlinguistic symbolic abilities in language-impaired children. *Journal of Speech and Hearing Disorders, 49,* 169–176.

Kamhi, A., & Koenig, L. (1985). Metalinguistic awareness in normal and language-disordered children. *Language, Speech, Hearing Services in Schools, 16,* 199–210.

Karmiloff-Smith, A. (1980). Psychological processes underlying pronominalization and non-pronominalization in children's connected discourse. In J. Kreiman & A.E. Ojeda (Eds.), *Papers from the parasession on pronouns and anaphora* (pp.231–250). Chicago: Chicago Linguistic Society.

Kellermann, K., Broetzmann, S., Lim, T., & Kitao, K. (1989). The conversation mop: Scenes in the stream of discourse. *Discourse Processes, 12,* 27–61.

Kintsch, W. (1974). *The representation of meaning in memory.* Hillsdale, NJ: Erlbaum.

Klein-Konigsberg, E. (1984). Semantic integration and language learning disabilities: From research to assessment and intervention. In G. P. Wallach & K. G. Butler (Eds.), *Language learning disabilities in school-age children* (pp. 251–270). Baltimore, MD: Williams & Wilkins.

Lahey, M. (1990). Who shall be called language disordered? Some reflections and one perspective. *Journal of Speech and Hearing Disorders, 36,* 612–620.

Liberman, I., & Shankweiller, D. (1985). Phonology and the problems of learning to read and write. *Remedial and Special Education, 6,* 8–17.

Liles, B.Z. (1993). Narrative discourse in children with language disorders and children with normal language: A critical review of the literature. *Journal of Speech and Hearing Research, 36,* 868–882.

Liles, B.Z. (1987). Episode organization and cohesive conjunctions in narratives of children with and without language disorder. *Journal of Speech and Hearing Research, 30,* 185–196.

Liles, B.Z. (1985). Cohesion in the narratives of normal and language disordered children. *Journal of Speech and Hearing Research, 28,* 123–133.

Lloyd, P. (1994). Referential communication: Assessment and intervention. *Topics in Language Disorders, 14,* 55–69.

Lloyd, P., Camaioni, L., & Ercolani, P. (in press). Assessing referential communication skills in the primary school years: A comparative study. *British Journal of Developmental Psychology.*

Lund, N., & Duchan, J. (1988). *Assessing children's language in naturalistic contexts.* Englewood Cliffs, NJ: Prentice–Hall.

Lundberg, I., Olofsson, A., & Wall, S. (1980). Reading and spelling skill in first school years predicted from phonemic awareness skills in kindergarten. *Scandinavian Journal of Psychology, 21,* 159–173.

Magnusson, E., & Nauclér, K. (1990). Reading and spelling in language-disordered children—linguistic and metalinguistic prerequisites: Report on a longitudinal study. *Clinical Linguistics and Phonetics, 4,* 49–61.

Mandler, J., & Johnson, N. (1977). Remembrance of things parsed: Story structure and recall. *Cognitive Psychology, 9,* 111–151.

McCabe, A., & Rollins, P. (1994). Assessment of preschool narrative skills. *American Journal of Speech-Language Pathology, 3,* 45–55.

McCauley, R., & Swisher, L. (1984). Use and misuse of norm-referenced tests in clinical assessment: A hypothetical case. *Journal of Speech and Hearing Disorders, 49,* 338–348.

McTear, M. (1985). *Children's conversation.* Oxford: Blackwell.

Mentis, M. (1994). Topic management in discourse: Assessment and intervention. *Topics in Language Disorders, 14,* 29–54.

Mentis, M., & Prutting, C. (1987). Cohesion in the discourse of normal and head-injured adults. *Journal of Speech and Hearing Research, 30,* 88–98.

Menyuk, P., Chesnick, M., Liebergott, J., Korngold, B., D'Agostino, R., & Belanger, A. (1991). Predicting reading problems in at-risk children. *Journal of Speech and Hearing Research, 34,* 893–903.

Merritt, D. S., & Liles, B. Z. (1987). Story grammar ability in children with and without language disorder: Story generation, story retelling, and story comprehension. *Journal of Speech and Hearing Research, 30,* 539–551.

Miller, L. (1990). The roles of language and learning in the development of literacy. *Topics in Language Disorders,10,* 1–24.

Miranda, E., McCabe, A., & Bliss, L. (1993). Jumping around and leaving things out. Manuscript submitted for publication.

Naremore, R. (1994). Story re-telling as an assessment tool. Manuscript submitted for publication.

Nelson, K. (Ed.). (1986). *Event knowledge: Structure and function in development.* Hillsdale, NJ: Erlbaum.

Nelson, K. (1981). Social cognition in a script framework. In J. H. Flavell & L. Ross (Eds.), *Social cognitive development: Frontier and possible futures.* New York, NY: Cambridge University Press.

Nelson, K. (1978). How young children represent knowledge in their world in and out of language. In R. S. Seigler (Ed.), *Children's thinking: What develops?* Hillsdale, NJ: Erlbaum.

Nelson, K., Fivush, R., Hudson, J., & Lucariello, J. (1983). Scripts and the development of memory. In M. T. H. Chi (Ed.), *Contributions to human development: Trends in memory development research (Vol.9).* New York, NY: Karger.

Nelson, K., & Gruendel, J. (1986). Children's scripts. In K. Nelson (Ed.), *Event knowledge: Structure and function in development.* Hillsdale, NJ: Erlbaum.

Nelson, K., & Gruendel, J. (1981). Generalized event representations: Basic building blocks of cognitive development. In A. Brown & M. Lamb (Eds.), *Advances in developmental psychology (Vol.1).* Hillsdale, NJ: Erlbaum.

Nesdale, A. R., Herriman, M. L., & Tunmer, W. E. (1984). Phonological awareness in children. In W. E. Tunmer, C. Pratt, & M. L. Herriman (Eds.), *Metalinguistic awareness in children: Theory, research and implications.* New York: Springer–Verlag.

Nye, C., and Montgomery, J.K. (1989). Identification criteria for language disordered children: A national survey. *Hearsay: The Journal of the Ohio Speech and Hearing Association,* Spring, 26–33.

Oakhill, J. (1984). Inferential and memory skills in children's comprehensions of stories. *British Journal of Educational Psychology, 54,* 31–39.

Postman, N. (1985). *Amusing ourselves to death.* New York: Viking Penguin.

Propp, V. (1958). The morphology of the folktale. *International Journal of American Linguistics, 4,* 1–134. (Originally published in Russian in 1928).

Purcell, S. L., & Liles, B. Z. (1992). Cohesion repairs in the narratives of normal-language and language-disordered school-age children. *Journal of Speech and Hearing Research, 35,* 354–362.

Rapin, I. (1987). Developmental dysphasia and autism in pre-school children: Characteristics and subtypes. In *Proceedings of the First International Symposium on Specific Speech and Language Disorders in Children.* London: AFASIC.

Rapin, I., & Allen, D. (1983). Developmental language disorders: Nosologic consideration. In U. Kirk (Ed.), *Neuropsychology of language, reading and spelling.* New York: Academic Press.

Rice, M. L., Sell, M. A., & Hadley, P. A. (1991). Social interactions of speech and language impaired children. *Journal of Speech and Hearing Research, 34,* 1299–1307.

Ripich, D. N., & Griffith, P. L. (1988). Narrative abilities of children with learning disabilities and nondisabled children: Story structure, cohesion, and propositions. *Journal of Learning Disabilities, 21,* 165–173.

Robinson, E. J., & Robinson, W. P. (1976). The young child's understanding of communication. *Developmental Psychology, 12,* 328–333.

Robinson, E. J., & Whittaker, S. (1987). Children's conceptions of relations between messages, meanings and reality. *British Journal of Developmental Psychology, 5,* 81–90.

Roseberry, C. A., & Connell, P. J. (1991). The use of an invented language rule in the differentiation of normal and language-impaired Spanish-speaking children. *Journal of Speech and Hearing Research, 34,* 596–603.

Rosinski-McClendon, M.K., & Newhoff, M. (1987). Conversational responsiveness and assertiveness in language impaired children. *Language, Speech, and Hearing Services in Schools, 18,* 53–62.

Ross, B. L., and Berg, C. A. (1990). Individual differences in script reports: Implications for language assessment. *Topics in Language Disorders, 10,* 30–44.

Roth, F. P., & Spekman, N. J. (1985). Story grammar analysis of narratives produced by learning disabled and normally achieving students. Paper presented at the Symposium on Research in Child Language Disorders, Madison, WI.

Rumelhart, D. (1977). Understanding and summarizing brief stories. In D. LaBerge & S. Jay (Eds.), *Basic processes in reading: Perception and comprehension.* Hillsdale, NJ: Lawrence Erlbaum Associates.

Rumelhart, D. (1975). Notes on a schema for stories. In D. Bobrow & A. Collins (Eds.), *Representation and understanding: Studies in cognitive science* (pp.211–236). New York: Academic Press.

Savich, P. (1980). *A comparison of the anticipatory imagery and spatial representation ability of normal and language disabled children.* Unpublished doctoral dissertation, University of Colorado, Boulder.

Saywitz, K. & Cherry-Wilkinson, L. (1982). Age-related differences in metalinguistic awareness. In S. Kuczaj (Ed.), *Language development: Vol. 2. Language, thought, and culture.* Hillsdale, NJ: Erlbaum.

Schank, R. C., & Abelson, R. P. (1977). *Scripts, plans, goals, and understanding.* Hillsdale, NJ: Erlbaum.

Semel, E., Wiig, E., & Secord, W. (1987). *Clinical Evaluation of Language Fundamentals—Revised.* Boston: The Psychological Corporation.

Slackman, E., Hudson, J., & Fivush, R. (1986). Actions, actors, links, and goals: The structure of children's event representation. In K. Nelson (Ed.), *Event knowledge: Structure and function in development.* Hillsdale, NJ: Erlbaum.

Smith, C., & Tager-Flusberg, H. (1982). Metalinguistic awareness and language development. *Journal of Experimental Psychology, 34*, 449–468.

Snyder, L. (1984). Developmental language disorders: Elementary school age. In A. Holland (Ed.), *Language disorders in children: Recent advances* (pp. 129–158). San Diego: College-Hill Press.

Sonnenschein, S., & Whitehurst, G. (1984). Developing referential communication: A hierarchy of skills. *Child Development, 55*, 1936–1945.

Sparrow, S., Balla, D., & Cicchetti, D. (1984). *Vineland Adaptive Behavior Scales.* Circle Pines, MN: American Guidance Service.

Spreen, O., & Haaf, R. G. (1986). Empirically derived LD subtypes: A replication attempt and longitudinal patterns over fifteen years. *Journal of Learning Disabilities, 19*, 170–180.

Stark, R., & Tallal, P. (1981). Selection of children with specific language deficits. *Journal of Speech and Hearing Disorders, 46*, 114–122.

Stein, N.L. (1979). How children understand stories: A developmental analysis. In L. Katz (Ed.), *Current topics in early childhood education*, Vol. 2, (pp.261–290). Norwood, NJ: Ablex.

Stein, N., & Glenn, C. (1979). An analysis of story comprehension in elementary school children. In R.O. Freedle (Ed.), *New directions in discourse processing.* Norwood, NJ: Ablex.

Stephens, M. I. & Montgomery, A. A. (1985). A critique of recent relevant standardized tests. *Topics in Language Disorders, 5*, 21–45.

Stoel-Gammon, C., & Hedberg, N. (1984). *A longitudinal study of cohesion in the narratives of young children.* Third International Congress for the Study of Child Language, Austin, TX.

Tallal, P., Curtiss, S., & Kaplan, R. (1989). *The San Diego longitudinal study: Evaluating the outcomes of preschool impairment in language development.* Final Report, NINCDS. Washington, DC.

Thorndyke, P. (1977). Cognitive structures in comprehension and memory. *Cognitive Psychology, 9*, 77–110.

Todorov, T. (1971). The two principles of narrative. *Diacritics, 1*, 37–44.

Torgeson, J., & Goldman, T. (1977). Rehearsal and short-term memory in second grade reading disabled children. *Child Development, 48*, 56–61.

Tunmer, W., & Bowey, J. (1984). Metalinguistic awareness and reading acquisition. In W. Tunmer, C. Pratt, & M. Herriman (Eds.), *Metalinguistic awareness in children: Theory, research, and implications.* New York: Springer-Verlag.

Tunmer, W., & Nesdale, A. (1985). Phoneme segmentation skill and beginning reading. *Journal of Educational Psychology, 77*, 417–427.

van Kleeck, A. (1982). The emergence of linguistic awareness: A cognitive framework. *Merrill-Palmer Quarterly, 28*, 237–265.

van Kleeck, A., & Bryant, D. (1984, November). Learning that language is arbitrary: Evidence from early lexical changes. Paper presented at the meeting of the American Speech-Language-Hearing Association, San Francisco.

van Kleeck, A., & Schuele, C.M. (1987). Precursors to literacy: normal development. *Topics in Language Disorders, 7*, 13–31.

Vygotsky, L.S. (1962). *Thought and language.* Cambridge, MA: MIT Press.

Wagner, R., & Torgesen, J. (1987). The nature of phonological processing and its causal role in the acquisition of reading skills. *Psychological Bulletin, 101,* 192–212.

Walker, H. M., Schwarz, I. E., Nippold, M. A., Irvin, L. K., Noell, J. W. (1994). Social skills in school-age children and youth: Issues and best practices in assessment and intervention. *Topics in Language Disorders, 14,* 70–82.

Wallach, G. P. (1990). Magic buries Celtics: Looking for broader interpretations of language learning and literacy. *Topics in Language Disorders, 10,* 63–80.

Wallach, G. P., & Liebergott, J. W. (1984). Who shall be called "learning disabled?": Some new directions. In G. P. Wallach and K. G. Butler (Eds.), *Language learning disabilities in school-age children.* Baltimore, MD: Williams and Wilkins.

Wallach, G., & Miller, L. (1988). *Language intervention and academic success.* Boston: College-Hill Press.

Weaver, P., & Dickinson, D. (1982). Scratching below the surface structure: Exploring the usefulness of story grammars. *Discourse Processes, 5,* 225–243.

Wells, G. (1985). *Language development in the pre-school years.* Cambridge: Cambridge University Press.

Wells, G. (1981). *Learning through interaction.* Cambridge: Cambridge University Press.

Westby, C. E. (1984). Development of narrative language abilities. In G. P. Wallach & K. G. Butler (Eds.), *Language learning disabilities in school-age children* (pp.103–127). Baltimore, MD: Williams & Wilkins.

Westby, C. E. (1982). Cognitive and linguistic aspects of children's narrative development. *Communicative Disorders,7,* 1–16.

Westby, C. E., Maggart, Z. & Van Dongen, R. (1984). Oral narratives of students varying in reading ability. Paper presented at the Third International Congress for the Study of Child Language. Austin, TX.

Westby, C. E., & Martinez, B. (1981). Facilitating narrative abilities in mid-school students. Paper presented at the American Speech-Language-Hearing Association Convention, Los Angeles, CA.

Wiig, E., & Semel, E. (1976). *Language disabilities in children and adolescents.* Columbus, OH: Merrill.

Zhurova, L. (1973). The development of analysis of words into their sounds by preschool children. In C.A. Ferguson & D.I. Slobin (Eds.), *Studies of child language development.* New York: Holt, Rinehart, & Winston.

A P P E N D I X   1

Cumulative Files:
Mitch and Jackie

MITCH

    Speech and Hearing Center Final Report
    Hearing Screening Form
    Kindergarten Report Card
    Student Assistance Team Referral Form
    Chapter I Profile Report
    Resource Teacher Observation Form
    Psychological Report

JACKIE

    Psychological Report
    End-of-Year Report: Second Grade
    Hearing Screening Form
    Student Assistance Team Referral Form

Cumulative File: Mitch

```
                    SEMESTER PROGRESS REPORT:
                    SUMMARY AND RECOMMENDATIONS

NAME: Mitch ---                  THERAPY PERIOD: 5/91-8/91
AGE: 6-5                         TOTAL HOURS: 21
BIRTHDATE: 3/4/85                CLINICIAN: Ann Webster
PARENT: Jean & David             SUPERVISOR: Betty Norris
ADDRESS 705 Bruce Ct.              M.A. CCC-SLP
     Madison, --                 DISORDER: Language
```

BACKGROUND INFORMATION:

Mitch has been enrolled in language intervention at this clinic
since the age of three years. This semester Mitch was enrolled in
individual treatment sessions twice a week for 45 minutes per
session.

SUMMARY OF INTERVENTION:

At the beginning of this semester, Mitch was observed to continue
to confuse the first person pronouns (me/I) and to be
inconsistent in his use of the "to be" verb in either an
auxiliary or copular usage. Mitch also demonstrated difficulty
converting known scripts into linguistic representations and also
lacked story structure as demonstrated in story re-telling.

Intervention stressed and used stories that emphasized the areas
of language form that Mitch required (pronouns, verb "to be").
Stories were also used to stress scripts and simple story
structures. At all stages of intervention, Mitch was asked to
retell the story and strategies and scaffolding were provided as
appropriate. The stories used contained a strong episodic
structure (only one episode per story) and were largely first
person accounts of a boy like Mitch. Books were created that
emphasized the scripts that Mitch was involved in such as "Going
to McDonalds", "Going to a Birthday Party", "Going to the Zoo".
Mitch was required to order the pictures and tell the clinician
what to write for each. Scaffolding and probes were provided to
elicit more that just a picture description. The books were sent
home so that Mitch could "read" the stories and scripts to his
family.

By the end of the summer session, Mitch used the appropriate
pronoun in all instances within the intervention session and was
heard to use it outside of the clinic as well. His use of the "to
be" verb was observed to be used appropriately in most
situations. His ability to relate a familiar script showed
improvement as long as he had the visual support of pictures to
guide him. His story retelling still required considerable
scaffolding from an adult.

RECOMMENDATIONS:

1. Since Mitch will be enrolled in kindergarten this fall no further treatment at this Center is recommended.

2. Mitch should be evaluated by his school Speech-Language Pathologist for enrollment in intervention. Intervention should focus on:
   a. story grammar as evidenced in story retelling
   b. scripting as evidenced in event retelling

3. The family is urged to continue to read to Mitch on a regular basis. They were provided with a list of books which stress either problem/solution structure or scripting.

Ann Webster
Graduate Clinician

Betty Norris, M.A. CCC-SLP
Clinical Associate Professor

School: _____   Date: _____

Teacher: _____   Grade: _1st_

Child's Name: _Mitch_

PARENT PERMISSION FORM

HEARING SCREENING

I request a hearing screening for _Mitch_.
                                 (child's name)

_____
                    Parent/Guardian

Your child's hearing will be screened by the Speech Language Pathologist. This is only a screening. You will be notified of the results once the screening has been completed. Failure to pass the screening will result in referral to a physician for further evaluation and treatment.

Thank You,

Marilyn

Speech Language Pathologist

All screenings are conducted at 20db unless otherwise noted.

	500 Hz	1000 Hz	2000 Hz	3000 Hz	4000 Hz	6000 Hz	8000 Hz
R	20	20	20	20	20	20	20
L	20	20	20	20	20	20	20

Remarks: _Mitch was also given an impedance test. He passed this test as well as the pure tone screening._

Kindergarten Report Card (Page 1)

NAME _Mitch_

SCHOOL _Trigg Elementary_

TEACHER _Sue Chandler_ YEAR _____

PRINCIPAL _Frank Thompson_

ATTENDANCE

	1	2	3	4
DAYS ABSENT	2	2	1	0
DAYS PRESENT	43	43	44	45

+ THE STUDENT HAS THE SKILL
O THE STUDENT USES THE SKILL MOST OF THE TIME
✓ THE STUDENT IS BEGINNING TO DEVELOP THE SKILL

SOCIAL AND EMOTIONAL DEVELOPMENT

TERM	2	3	4
EXPRESSES HIS/HER NEEDS			
TAKES TURNS, WORKS AND PLAYS WELL WITH OTHERS	✓	O	+
TAKES CARE OF PERSONAL BELONGINGS	✓	+	+
CLEANS UP AND PUTS THINGS AWAY	✓	+	+
MEETS NEW EXPERIENCES WITH CONFIDENCE	✓	+	+
RESPECTS THE RIGHTS OF OTHERS	✓	+	+
ACCEPTS LIMITS ON ACTIVITIES, SPACE AND MATERIALS	✓	+	+
TAKES PRIDE IN WORK AND ACHIEVEMENTS	✓	+	+
WORKS WITHOUT DISTURBING OTHERS	✓	O	O
CHOOSES VARIETY OF ACTIVITIES	✓	O	+
ADAPTS TO CHANGES IN ROUTINE, SCHEDULE AND ROOM ARRANGEMENT	✓	O	O

PHYSICAL DEVELOPMENT: FINE MOTOR

TERM	2	3	4
HOLDS PENCIL AND CRAYON CORRECTLY	✓	+	+
CAN BUTTON, ZIP, AND SNAP	✓	+	+
CAN TRACE NEATLY	✓	+	+
CAN TIE			+
CAN COPY SHAPES AND LETTERS			+
CAN CUT WITH EASE AND SKILL			+
CAN PASTE OR GLUE NEATLY			+

PHYSICAL DEVELOPMENT: GROSS MOTOR

TERM	2	3	4
MOVES PARTS OF BODY FREELY	+	+	+
CAN HOP ON ONE FOOT		+	+
CAN JUMP FORWARD		+	+
CAN THROW AND CATCH		+	+
CAN WALK ON BALANCE BEAM			+
CAN SKIP			+

Kindergarten Report Card (Page 2)

FACTORS IMPORTANT IN ACADEMIC PROGRESS

TERM	2	3	4
PARTICIPATES IN DISCUSSIONS	✓	o	o
USES COMPLETE SENTENCES	o	+	+
SUSTAINS INTEREST IN AN ACTIVITY	o	o	+
ABLE TO WORK IN LARGE AND SMALL GROUP SETTINGS	✓	o	+
BEGINS AND COMPLETES ASSIGNED TASK	✓	✓	✓
FOLLOWS TWO OR MORE DIRECTIONS *needs work here. No progress*			
RECOGNIZES EIGHT BASIC COLORS	+	+	+
RECOGNIZES FOUR BASIC SHAPES	+	+	+
RECOGNIZES NUMERALS 0-9	+	+	+
COUNTS TO *30*	+	+	+
WRITES NUMBERS TO *10*	+	+	+
RECOGNIZES FIRST NAME IN PRINT	o	o	+
RECOGNIZES LAST NAME IN PRINT	✓	✓	✓
DRAWS PICTURE OF COMPLETE PERSON	+	+	+
IDENTIFIES UPPER CASE LETTERS		✓	✓
WRITES FIRST NAME		✓	+
RECOGNIZES AND COMPLETES PATTERN		✓	✓
UNDERSTANDS AND DEMONSTRATES ONE-TO-ONE CORRESPONDENCE		✓	o
CORRECTLY SEQUENCES 2,3,4,5 NUMBERS		✓	o
CORRECTLY SEQUENCES PICTURES AND EVENTS		✓	✓
CAN SORT OBJECTS BY COLOR, SHAPE, SIZE, CATEGORY		✓	✓
CAN APPROPRIATELY ASK WHO, WHAT, WHERE, WHEN, WHY QUESTIONS		+	+
UNDERSTANDS THE CONCEPT OF OPPOSITE			✓
INDENTIFIES EIGHT BASIC COLORS			+
IDENTIFIES FOUR BASIC SHAPES			+
IDENTIFIES NUMERALS 0-9			+
WRITES LAST NAME			o
IDENTIFIES LOWER CASE LETTERS			✓
IDENTIFIES CONSONANT SOUNDS *needs work.*			
CAN COMPLETE A RHYMING PHRASE *needs work – inconsistent*			
RECOGNIZES SOUNDS AT THE BEGINNING AND END OF WORDS *NO !*			
IS DEVELOPING A BASIC READING VOCABULARY *NO !*			
IS DEVELOPING A PERSONAL READING VOCABULARY *NO !*			

COMMENTS

Second Grading Period *no progress w/ phonics*   Fourth Grading Period *no progress with phonics*

Third Grading Period *no progress in phonics or reading*

GRADE ASSIGNMENT

Promoted to *1st*

Retained in _____

Teacher's Signature *Sue Chandler*

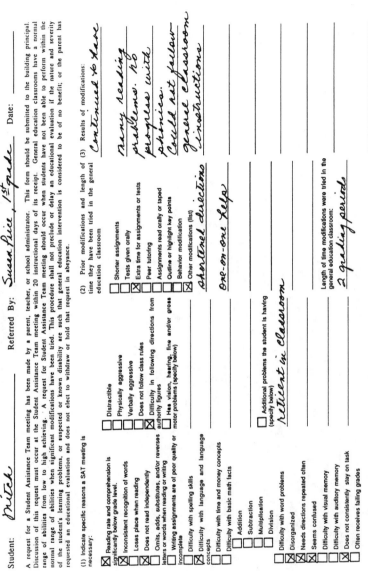

Request For Student Assistance Team Meeting

Student: _Mitch_   Referred By: _Susan Price, 1st grade_   Date:

A request for a Student Assistance Team meeting has been made by a parent, teacher, or school administrator. This form should be submitted to the building principal. Discussion of this request must occur at the Student Assistance Team meeting within 20 instructional days of its receipt. General education classrooms have a normal range of abilities from low to high achieving. A request for Student Assistance Team meeting should occur when students have not been able to perform within the normal range of abilities when significant modifications have been tried. This procedure shall not preclude or delay an educational evaluation if the nature and severity of the student's learning problems, or suspected or known disability are such that general education intervention is considered to be of no benefit; or the parent has requested an educational evaluation and does not elect to withdraw or hold that request in abeyance.

(1) Indicate specific reasons a SAT meeting is necessary:

- ☒ Reading rate and comprehension is significantly below grade level.
- ☒ Inconsistent recognition of words
- ☐ Loses place when reading
- ☒ Does not read independently
- ☐ Omits, adds, substitutes, and/or reverses letters or words when reading or writing
- ☐ Writing assignments are of poor quality or incomplete
- ☐ Difficulty with spelling skills
- ☒ Difficulty with language and language concepts
- ☐ Difficulty with time and money concepts
- ☐ Difficulty with basic math facts
  - ☐ Addition
  - ☐ Subtraction
  - ☐ Multiplication
  - ☐ Division
- ☐ Difficulty with word problems
- ☒ Disorganized
- ☒ Needs directions repeated often
- ☒ Seems confused
- ☐ Difficulty with visual memory
- ☐ Difficulty with auditory memory
- ☒ Does not consistently stay on task
- ☐ Often receives failing grades

- ☐ Distractible
- ☐ Physically aggressive
- ☐ Verbally aggressive
- ☐ Does not follow class rules
- ☒ Difficulty in following directions from authority figures
- ☐ Has vision, hearing, fine and/or gross motor problems (specify below)

_____

- ☐ Additional problems the student is having (specify below)
Reticent in classroom

(2) Prior modifications and length of time they have been tried in the general education classroom

- ☐ Shorter assignments
- ☐ Tests given orally
- ☒ Extra time for assignments or tests
- ☐ Peer tutoring
- ☐ Assignments read orally or taped
- ☐ Outline or highlight key points
- ☐ Behavior modification
- ☒ Other modifications (list)
shortned directions
one-on-one help

Length of time modifications were tried in the general education classroom:
2 grading periods

(3) Results of modifications:
Continued to have
many reading
problems. no
progress with
phonics.
Could not follow
general classroom
instructions

White-Director   Canary- Parents   Pink- School   Gold - School Psych. ⸗

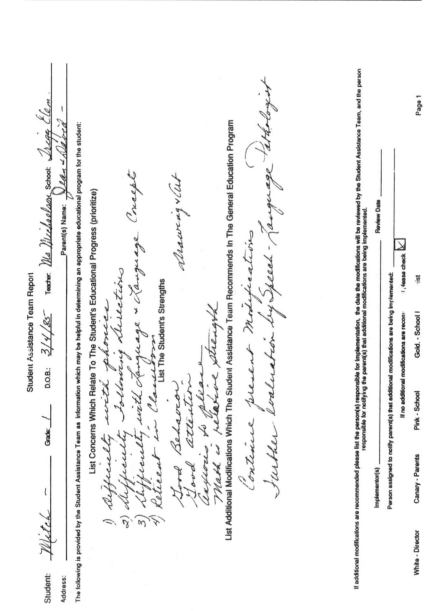

Student Assistance Team Report

Student: _Mitch_ —   Grade: _1_   D.O.B.: _3/4/85_   Teacher: _Ms. Nicholson_ School: _Bragg Elem._

Address: _____   Parent(s) Name: _Jean David_ —

The following is provided by the Student Assistance Team as information which may be helpful in determining an appropriate educational program for the student:

List Concerns Which Relate To The Student's Educational Progress (prioritize)

1) difficulty with phonics
2) difficulty following directions
3) difficulty with language & language concepts
4) reticent in classroom

List The Student's Strengths

Good Behavior
Good attention
Enjoys to please   drawing/art
Math is relative strength

List Additional Modifications Which The Student Assistance Team Recommends In The General Education Program

Continue present modifications
Further Evaluation by Speech-Language Pathologist

If additional modifications are recommended please list the person(s) responsible for implementation, the date the modifications will be reviewed by the Student Assistance Team, and the person responsible for notifying the parent(s) that additional modifications are being implemented.

Implementor(s) _____   Review Date _____

Person assigned to notify parent(s) that additional modifications are being implemented: _____

If no additional modifications are recommended, please check ☒

White - Director   Canary - Parents   Pink - School   Gold. - School List

Page 1

Student Assistance Team Report

Date: _____

Student: _Mitch_ - _____

The Student Assistance Team has reviewed the following information regarding the student's educational history:

☒ SE 1 (Request For Student Assistance Team Meeting)

☒ The student's educational history

☒ The student's strengths and weaknesses

☒ The feasibility of additional modifications in the general education program

☐ Additional Information (specify) _____

The Student Assistance Team , after reviewing the information specified above, makes the following recommendation(s):

☐ Continue general education with program modifications

☒ Refer to a multi-disciplinary evaluation team for an educational evaluation to determine the presence of a possible disability which may be affecting educational performance

☐ Refer to a multi-disciplinary evaluation team for mandatory three year re-evaluation for continued eligibility for special education

☐ Other (specify) _____

If the Student Assistance Team makes a referral to a multi-disciplinary evaluation team the following appointments are made:

Person assigned as the student's Case Conference Coordinator: _Mr. Thorzhuer_

Multi-Disciplinary Evaluation Team Members:

Person assigned to obtain parent permission for evaluation: _Martha Grayson / Martha Grayson_

Person assigned to obtain a social / developmental history: _Martha Grayson / Kathy Trahn_

School psychologist: _Mr. Michaelson_

Special education teacher:

(must be licensed in suspected disability area)

General education teacher: _Wasielzy_

Other specialist(s): _____

Student Assistance Team Members:
(sign below)

Martha Grayson
Martha Grayson

Kathy Trahn
Mr. Michaelson

White - Director   Canary - Parents   Pink - School   Gold - School Psychologist

CHAPTER I PROFILE

Name _Mitch_

School _Trigg Elementary_ Grade _1st_ Classroom Teacher _Miss Michaelson_

Chapter I Assistant _Susan Osborn_

Diagnostic Test Results Fall of _19___

Total Percent _18%_

Comments _Mitch performed below grade level in_
both reading (decoding) and reading comprehension

Vocabulary Achievement in Basal Reader

Level _primer_ _12_ %

Level _____ _____ %

Level _____ _____ %

Level _____ _____ %

Number of books read in Chapter I FY ___ _10_

Standardized Test Scores

Test _Gates-McGinitie_   Date administered _December_

Vocabulary : _____ NCE _____ Percentile

Comprehension: _____ NCE _____ Percentile

Total Reading: _1_ NCE _2ND_ Percentile

Did student attend Chapter I prior to this school year? _NO_

If so, how many years has student attended Chapter I classes? _____

Was student referred in the spring of last year for Chapter I Screening? _YES_

If not, how/when was student selected for Chapter I services? _____

Behavioral items checked below have been observed in Chapter I services.

Student strengths _good behavior, good attention, cooperative,_

Low self esteem _no_

Short attention span _no_

Completing work _if given enough time and good, clear directions_

Listening _good_

Additional comments _Mitch appears to do best using a_
whole word approach to instruction. He always
enjoys thinking of a theme to study.

Educational Evaluation / Observation Report Form

STUDENT: *Mitch*   D.O.B.: *3/4/85*

DATE(S) OF OBSERVATION: _____

SCHOOL: _____ GRADE: *1* HOME SCHOOL CORP: _____

TEACHER CONDUCTING OBSERVATION (must be licensed in area of suspected disability): *Kathy Trahan*

1.   FORMAL TESTS ADMINISTERED (IF ANY):

_____

2.   RESULTS OF TESTS / OBSERVATION:

Having difficulty with phonics. Does not follow directions well — depends on watching other children. Observed during reading class. Could not identify beginning & ending sounds. Never raised his hand. Seemed confused about story content. Could not relate own experiences to story

3.   RECOMMENDATIONS:

Refer to case conference committee for discussion.

_____

SIGNATURE OF TEACHER CONDUCTING OBSERVATION: *Kathy Trahan*

POSITION: *LD Resource Teacher*

AREA(S) OF CERTIFICATION: *Special Ed / LD*   DATE: _____

This form must be completed for students suspected of having disabilities in the following area(s):
Dual sensory impairment, emotional handicap, learning disability, visual impairment.
Also, any student entering Early Childhood special education and, as appropriate in other disability categories, need to have documentation of an observation by a teacher licensed in the area of suspected disability.

White - Director   Canary - Parents   Pink - School

EDUCATIONAL EVALUATION

School District: XXXXXXXXXXXXXXX   School: XXXXXXXX Elementary

Child's Name: Mitch
Sex: M
Date of Birth: 3/4/85
Age: 8-1

Grade: 1st
Parent(s):Jean & David
Address: 705 Bruce Ct.
Madison

Tests Administered and Results: Date of Test: March 15, 199_
Wechsler Intelligence Scale for Children-Revised (WISC-R)

Bender Visual Motor Gestalt Test (B-G)

Peabody Picture Vocabulary Test-Revised (PPVT-R), Form M

Kaufman Test of Educational Achievement (K*TEA), Comprehensive Form

Review of Records

Reason for Referral:

Mitch was referred for evaluation of his academic ability and determination of
eligibility for Special Education Services.

Background Information:

Mitch is an 8 year, 1 month old male currently enrolled in first grade at XXXXXXXXX
Elementary School. The referral for evaluation, completed by his first grade teacher,
indicates that he is experiencing difficulty with reading mechanics and comprehension,
written expression, math reasoning, and expressive language. Mitch was held out of
kindergarten 1 year due to delays in communication skills, and thus has age advantage
in his current grade placement.

No history of hearing difficulties was reported. Recent hearing screening yielded
normal results. No history of vision problems was reported. In general, no health
concerns were indicated.

During the testing sessions, Mitch was cooperative with all Examiner requests. He did, however, require a great deal of encouragement in order to persist as the test became difficult. He made several negative self-statements such as, "I can't do this", throughout the evaluation. Mitch tended to work quickly and, at times, haphazardly on Performance Scale items. In general, rapport was adequately established and the current test results are judged to be a valid estimate of Mitch's present functioning levels.

Test Results:

Wechsler Intelligence Test For Children - Revised

The WISC-R is an individually administered test which results in a general intelligence quotient or learning rate. The student performs a variety of tasks (subtests) which are normed at age.

The test is divided into verbal and nonverbal tasks. Each subtest on the Verbal Scale portion of the test requires listening and verbal expression. The Performance Scale involves visual-perceptual-motor skills, and these subtests are timed.

VERBAL   Scaled Scores

Information	7	-Memory of general information gained from experience and education.
Similarities	4	-Ability to see associational relationships and perform logical and abstract thinking.
Arithmetic	8	-Concentration, numerical concepts and basic math operations.
Vocabulary	8	-Word knowledge acquired from experience and education, kind and quality of language, and level of abstract thinking.
Comprehension	5	-Practical knowledge and judgement in social situations.
Digit Span	6	-Attention span, concentration, immediate auditory memory sequencing.

PERFORMANCE

Picture Completion	9	-Visual memory for common object, attention to detail.
Picture Arrangement	10	-Cause/effect relationships, visual

		sequencing, attention to details.
Block Design	7	-Reproduction of abstract designs, visual motor spatial coordination.
Object Assembly	5	-Ability to see part-whole relationships, visual motor spatial coordination.
Coding	8	-Paper/pencil task which requires visual motor integration.
(Mazes)	--	-Planning and foresight, pencil control, and visual-motor coordination.

Severely Deficient	Deficient	Below Average	Average	Above Average	Superior	Very Superior
1 2 3	4 5 6	7 8	9 10 11	12 13	14 15 16	17 18 19

Verbal Scale IQ: 78   Performance Scale IQ: 85   Full Scale IQ: 80
Wechsler Classification: Low Average   Percentile: 9

Comments: Mitch's overall cognitive ability, as measured by the WISC-R, appears to be in the low average range of global intelligence (FS IQ = 80 + /-6). The chances are 95 out of 100 that Mitch's true IQ fall within the range of scores from 74 to 86. Verbal and Performance Scale scores appear equally developed.

On the Verbal Scale section of the test, which is closely correlated with academic success, Mitch demonstrated below average ability on tasks measuring his general fund of information, numerical reasoning, and word knowledge. Specific weaknesses were noted in abstract reasoning ability, understanding of social situations presented verbally, and short-term auditory memory.

On the performance scale section of the test, which consists of visual and manual tasks, Mitch demonstrated adequate ability on those tasks requiring alertness to visual detail, and sequencing ability. Mitch scored in the below average range on items involving construction of a design by using a pattern, and short-term visual memory and visual motor speed. A weakness was also noted on a task requiring assembly of a whole from its component parts.

Bender Visual-Motor Gestalt Test

The Bender Visual-Motor Gestalt Test is a series of geometric forms which are copied onto blank paper and organized by the student. This test measures the integration of visual perceptual-motor and organizational skills through a paper and pencil task.

Raw Score: 11 Standard Score: 59 Age Equivalent: 5-4 to 5-5
Percentile: below 5

Comments: Mitch's performance on this test indicates that his perceptual motor and organizational skills are an area of weakness. He made numerous errors in distortion and integration of the figures. These weaknesses suggest that Mitch may experience difficulty with paper/pencil tasks, in copying information from the board, and on worksheets.

Peabody Picture Vocabulary Test - Revised

The PPVT-R is a test measuring receptive vocabulary skills. The student is given a word orally and he responds by selecting the picture which best illustrates the meaning of the stimulus word. There is no reading or verbal expression required.

Raw Score: 73   Standard Score: 76   Percentile: 5th
Age Equivalent: 6-3   Stanine: 2

Comments: Mitch's performance on this test suggests that his receptive vocabulary skills are at approximately the 6 year, 3 month level. This represents approximately a two year delay in comparison with his chronological age, but is commensurate with his verbal ability as measured by the WISC-R.

The Kaufman Test of Educational Achievement

The K*TEA is an individually administered measure of school achievement of children and adolescents in the first through twelfth grades.

Subtests	Grade Equivalent Score	Standard Score	Percentile Rank
Mathematics Applications	1.1	79	8
Reading Decoding	1.4	79	8
Spelling	1.4	78	7
Reading Comprehension	1.0	72	3
Mathematics Computation:	1.5	80	5

Composite Scales

Reading	1.2	75	5
Mathematics	1.3	79	8
Battery Composite	1.3	75	5

Comments: Mitch scored consistently at the beginning first grade level in all areas of achievement. His reading decoding skills are poor. He appears to utilize a sight word approach to reading. When encouraged to sound words out, he responded with, "I can't sound words out." Most of his decoding errors were in the form of word substitutions involving beginning letter sounds. His reading comprehension is measured at the pre-first grade level, with him unable to complete any items due to weak decoding skills. Spelling is also an area of weakness. Mitch spelled (4) out of (15) words presented. Again, he appeared to utilize a sight word approach to spelling words with little reliance on phonetic analysis. In Mathematics, Mitch was able to perform simple addition and subtraction problems, utilizing his fingers for counting. He did not appear to understand the concept of "carrying" for two-place addition problems.

In summary, Mitch's achievement in Reading, Spelling, and Mathematics appears commensurate with his overall ability as measured. His Achievement profile is characteristic of a slow learner.

Recommendations:

1. The Case Conference Committee should meet to review all evaluation data and decide upon appropriate educational programming.

2. Mitch should continue to be seen for speech and language therapy.

Martha Grayson
School Psychologist

Cumulative File: Jackie

```
                        PSYCHOEDUCATIONAL REPORT
Name:  Jackie--                 Parent: Karen & Kevin
D.O.B: 12/21/84                 Address: 17 Sherbrook Dr.
Age: 8-0                                 Springfield,--
Date Seen: 12/14/92             School: Westbrook
Grade: 2nd
```

Notes:

Jackie was referred for psychoeducational evaluation to rule out
a suspected learning disability.

There were no problems reported with pregnancy or delivery.
Developmental milestones were achieved on time. Jackie has never
suffered any serious illness or diseases.

Vision and hearing are reportedly within normal limits. Vision
and hearing appeared adequate for evaluation purposes.

Procedures Used:

Wechsler Intelligence Scale for Children-III (WISC-III)
Kaufman Test of Educational Achievement (K-TEA)
Bender-Visual Motor Gestalt Test
Learning Disability Evaluation Scale
Analytical Reading Inventory

Jackie achieved the following WISC-III IQ scores:
Verbal   76 (plus or minus 4)
Performance   107 (plus or minus 5)
Full Scale   90 (plus or minus 4)

Jackie's Full Scale score places her in the average range of
overall intelligence surpassing 25% of her age mates. Comparison
of Verbal vs. Performance scores suggests that Jackie performed
significantly better on nonverbal, less school related items,
than on verbal tasks requiring the use of language. While
Jackie's performance skills were measured at the upper end of the
average range, her verbal skills were in the borderline range.
This difference is sometimes indicative of a learning disability
and may also indicate the presents of a psycho-neurological
deficit.

On the Verbal Scale section of the test, which is closely
correlated with academic success, Jackie scored in the average
range on a task measuring short term auditory memory. Below
average ability was observed in abstract reasoning and numerical
reasoning. General knowledge, word knowledge and practical
judgement were all measured weaknesses for Jackie.

On the Performance Scale section of the test, which consists of
both visual and manual tasks, Jackie scored in the above average
range in alertness to visual detail, visual spatial relations and
visual processing speed. Average ability was observed in short

term visual memory and visual sequencing skills.

In general, these tests reflect overall average ability, with a significant preference for a visual presentation of information to which Jackie could respond manually. · Jackie's performance would suggest that she could be expected to perform academically at a level similar to same age peers. Because Jackie's leaning ability falls within the average range she meets one element of the LD criteria.

Achievement Factors:

Jackie achieved the following age based standard score equivalencies and percentiles on the K-TEA as administered by this examiner:

Mathematics Applications	88 (21st percentile)
Reading Decoding	81 (10th percentile)
Spelling	81 (10th percentile)
Reading Comprehension	85 (16th percentile)
Mathematics Computation	87 (19th percentile)
Reading Composite	82 (12th percentile)
Mathematics Composite	87 (19th percentile)
Battery Composite	82 (12th percentile)

(See standard score profile attached)

Jackie was administered the Analytical Reading Inventory as an additional measure of reading skills and obtained the following scores:

Grade	Word Lists	Estimated Levels	
Primer	55%	Independent	Not Obtained
First	20%	Instructional	Primer
		Frustration	First

When one considers Jackie's measured ability utilizing standard regression tables there is a severe discrepancy between expected and actual achievement levels in basic reading skills and written language.

No exclusionary factors have been demonstrated or documented in any area.

The Bender-Visual Motor Gestalt Test was administered as a screening of Jackie's visual motor and organizational skills. She obtained an age equivalent score of 11 years 0 months to 11 years 11 months. Her performance on this test suggests that these skills are well developed and that she should be able to handle most copying tasks in the classroom successfully.

Conclusions and Recommendations:

Jackie appears to meet eligibility requirements for placement in a learning disabilities program. However it should be noted that all placement decisions are to be made by the case conference committee after consideration of available information.

Ruth Ann Ballard
School Psychologist

TEST RESULTS

Wechsler Intelligence Scale for Children-III (68% confidence
levels for her age group reported)

Verbal   76 + or - 4
Performance   107 + or - 5
Full Scale   90 + or - 4

Verbal Subtests   Performance Subtest

Information   4   Picture Completion 12
Similarities   8   Picture Arrangement 11
Arithmetic   7   Block Design   12
Vocabulary   5   Object Assembly   11
Comprehension   5   Coding   9
Digit Span   9   Symbol Search   12

The Wechsler Scales have an average score of 10 and a standard
deviation of 3. Thus, scores of 7 or below are significantly
below the mean and scores of 13 and above are significantly above
the mean.

Kaufman Test of Educational Achievement (K-TEA)

	Standard Score	Grade Score	Percentile Score
Mathematics Applications	88	1.6	21
Reading Decoding	81	1.4	10
Spelling	81	1.4	10
Reading Comprehension	85	1.6	16
Mathematics Computation	87	1.6	19
Reading Composite	82	1.5	12
Mathematics Composite	87	1.6	19
Battery Composite	82	1.5	12

SECOND GRADE END OF YEAR SUMMARY
1990-1991 School Year/

Teacher: *Mrs. Day*   Student: *Jackie*

These are pieces of your WHOLE CHILD pulled apart and listed in isolation for the purpose of this evaluative summary (much like a disassembled puzzle). Second grade skills have been broken down in order to show strengths and weaknesses. It is important to look at these skills as they relate to your COMPLETE ASSEMBLED CHILD.

Skill Area	Mastery	OK	Weak

Phonetic Structural Analysis
  –vowel usage in various forms
  –consonant usuage in various forms
			✓

Vocabulary			✓

Story Elements
  main idea, details, sequence, setting, characterization,
  plot, making predictions, drawing conclusions, summarizing
			✓

Dictionary Usage ABC order, Glossaries			✓

Making Judgements
  fantasy/reality, classifying, making comparisons, cause
  and effect, context clues
			✓

Spelling Changes y to i, fe to v, dropping final e, doubling final consonant,			✓
Irregular Plurals		✓	
Contractions			✓
Syllable Division			✓
Homophones			✓
Suffixes and Prefixes			✓
Referents			✓

MATH AREAS AND NARRATIVE ON PAGE TWO

SECOND GRADE END OF YEAR SUMMARY   PAGE TWO

Student:

Skill Area			Firm Mastery	OK	Weak
Addition					
easy	count on	with carrying			
2 +5	12 + 6	589 + 346		✓	
Subtraction					
easy	count back	with borrowing			
8 −3	17 − 4	632 −379		✓	
Telling Time to the Minute					✓
Counting Money					✓
Problem Solving					✓
Place Value					✓

NARRATIVE:

Jackie is a talkative, friendly little girl. She has trouble telling organized stories. She seems to get lost in the middle of telling them. Her reading and written language are weak. Jackie seldom volunteers in class.

Jackie is very popular with her peer group. She is always neat in appearance and takes pride in her work.

_____   _____
Parent Signature   Date

School: _Trigg_   Date: _____

Teacher: _Mrs. Fulton_   Grade: _3rd_

Child's Name: _Jackie._

PARENT PERMISSION FORM

HEARING SCREENING

I request a hearing screening for _____.
                                           (child's name)

_____
                        Parent/Guardian

    Your child's hearing will be screened by the Speech Language
Pathologist. This is only a screening. You will be notified of
the results once the screening has been completed. Failure to pass
the screening will result in referral to a physician for further
evaluation and treatment.

                        Thank You,

                        Speech Language Pathologist

    All screenings are conducted at 20db unless otherwise noted.

	500 Hz	1000 Hz	2000 Hz	3000 Hz	4000 Hz	6000 Hz	8000 Hz
R	✓	✓	✓		✓		
L	✓	✓	✓		✓		

Remarks: _Pass_ _____

_____

_____

_____

Request For Student Assistance Team Meeting

Student: _Jackie_   Referred By: _Kathy Trahan_   Date: _____

A request for a Student Assistance Team meeting has been made by a parent, teacher, or school administrator. This form should be submitted to the building principal. Discussion of this request must occur at the Student Assistance Team meeting within 20 instructional days of its receipt. General education classrooms have a normal range of abilities from low to high achieving. A request for Student Assistance Team meeting should occur when students have not been able to perform within the normal range of abilities when significant modifications have been tried. This procedure shall not preclude or delay an educational evaluation if the nature and severity of the student's learning problems, or suspected or known disability are such that general education intervention is considered to be of no benefit; or the parent has requested an educational evaluation and does not elect to withdraw or hold that request in abeyance.

(1) Indicate specific reasons a SAT meeting is necessary:

- ☑ Reading rate and comprehension is significantly below grade level.
- ☐ Inconsistent recognition of words
- ☐ Loses place when reading
- ☐ Does not read independently
- ☐ Omits, adds, substitutes, and/or reverses letters or words when reading or writing
- ☑ Writing assignments are of poor quality or incomplete
- ☑ Difficulty with spelling skills
- ☐ Difficulty with language and language concepts
- ☐ Difficulty with time and money concepts
- ☐ Difficulty with basic math facts
  - ☐ Addition
  - ☐ Subtraction
  - ☐ Multiplication
  - ☑ Division
- ☑ Difficulty with word problems
- ☐ Disorganized
- ☑ Needs directions repeated often
- ☑ Seems confused
- ☐ Difficulty with visual memory
- ☑ Difficulty with auditory memory
- ☐ Does not consistently stay on task
- ☐ Often receives failing grades

- ☐ Distractible
- ☐ Physically aggressive
- ☐ Verbally aggressive
- ☐ Does not follow class rules
- ☐ Difficulty in following directions from authority figures
- ☐ Has vision, hearing, fine and/or gross motor problems (specify below)

none

☑ Additional problems the student is having (specify below)

Jackie often seems to know what she wants to say but has a hard time saying it when called on.

(2) Prior modifications and length of time they have been tried in the general education classroom

- ☐ Shorter assignments
- ☐ Tests given orally
- ☐ Extra time for assignments or tests
- ☐ Peer tutoring
- ☐ Assignments read orally or taped
- ☐ Outline or highlight key points
- ☑ Behavior modification
- ☑ Other modifications (list)

I try to give Jackie more time to respond.

Length of time modifications were tried in the general education classroom:

Since involvement in September.

(3) Results of modifications:

This doesn't seem to help.

Canary - Parents   Pink - School   Gold - School Psychologist

White - Director

Student Assistance Team Report

Student: _Jackie_____ Grade: _3_ D.O.B.: _____ Teacher: _____ School: _____

Address: _____ Parent(s) Name: _____

The following is provided by the Student Assistance Team as information which may be helpful in determining an appropriate educational program for the student:

List Concerns Which Relate To The Student's Educational Progress (prioritize)

Reading rate and comprehension (resource help)
Word finding
Difficulty expressing ideas
Seldom volunteers in class

List The Student's Strengths

Self-confident, friendly

List Additional Modifications Which The Student Assistance Team Recommends In The General Education Program

Allow more time to respond in class
Give her either/or choices to questions

If additional modifications are recommended please list the person(s) responsible for implementation, the date the modifications will be reviewed by the Student Assistance Team, and the person responsible for notifying the parent(s) that additional modifications are being implemented.

Implementor(s) _Classroom teacher/Resource teacher_ Review Date _____

Person assigned to notify parent(s) that additional modifications are being implemented: _____

If no additional modifications are recommended please check ☐

White - Director   Canary - Parents   Pink - School   Gold - School Psychologist

Page 1

Student Assistance Team Report

Date: _____

Student: _Jackie_

The Student Assistance Team has reviewed the following information regarding the student's educational history:

☒ SE 1 (Request For Student Assistance Team Meeting)

☒ The student's educational history

☒ The student's strengths and weaknesses

☒ The feasibility of additional modifications in the general education program

☐ Additional information (specify) _____

The Student Assistance Team , after reviewing the information specified above, makes the following recommendation(s):

☐ Continue general education with program modifications

☒ Refer to a multi-disciplinary evaluation team for an educational evaluation to determine the presence of a possible disability which may be affecting educational performance

☐ Refer to a multi-disciplinary evaluation team for mandatory three year re-evaluation for continued eligibility for special education

☐ Other (specify) _____

If the Student Assistance Team makes a referral to a multi-disciplinary evaluation team the following appointments are made:

Person assigned as the student's Case Conference Coordinator: _Mr. Thompson_

Person assigned to obtain parent permission for evaluation: _Martha Grayson_

Person assigned to obtain a social / developmental history: _Martha Grayson_

Multi-Disciplinary Evaluation Team Members:

School psychologist: _Martha Grayson_

Special education teacher: _Kathy Fraker_

(must be licensed in suspected disability area)

General education teacher: _Lori Martin_

Other specialist(s): _Marilyn_

White - Director   Canary - Parents   Pink - School   Gold - School Psychologist

Student Assistance Team Members:
(sign below)

_____
_____
_____
_____
_____

Page 2

Educational Evaluation / Observation Report Form

STUDENT: _Jackie_   D.O.B.: _12-21-84_

DATE(S) OF OBSERVATION: _Fall_

SCHOOL: _Trigg Elementary_ GRADE: _3_ HOME SCHOOL CORP: _____

TEACHER CONDUCTING OBSERVATION   _Kathy Trahan_

1.   FORMAL TESTS ADMINISTERED (IF ANY):

none

2.   RESULTS OF TESTS / OBSERVATION:

Jackie is a lively, friendly, self confident little girl. She seems to have difficulty expressing her ideas. She seldom volunteers to answer questions in class. She appears to have difficulty remembering what is said to her.

3.   RECOMMENDATIONS:

Refer Jackie to the Speech Language Pathologist for evaluation.

SIGNATURE OF TEACHER CONDUCTING OBSERVATION: _Kathy Trahan_

POSITION: _LRC teacher_

AREA(S) OF CERTIFICATION: _Special Education_ DATE: _____

This form must be completed for students suspected of having disabilities in the following area(s):
Dual sensory impairment, emotional handicap, learning disability, visual impairment.
Also, any student entering Early Childhood special education and, as appropriate in other disability categories, need to have documentation of an observation by a teacher
licensed in the area of suspected disability.

White - Director   Canary - Parents   Pink - School

Page 1 of 1

A P P E N D I X 2

Descriptions of Commercially Available Tests

Columbia Mental Maturity Scale. (1972). Burgemeister, B., Blum, L., & Lorge, I. New York: Harcourt Brace Jovanovich, Inc.

> The test yields an estimate of the general reasoning ability of children 3 years, 6 months through 9 years, 11 months in age. The test is easily administered, requiring no understanding of language beyond the word "different." Administration takes 15–20 minutes, including items designed to teach the child the task. Raw scores can be converted to get an estimate of performance IQ.

Clinical Evaluation of Language Fundamentals—Revised (CELF-R). (1987). Semel, E., Wiig, E., & Secord, W. San Antonio, TX: The Psychological Corporation

> The test battery includes eleven subtests for measuring syntax, semantics, and memory. The subtests are as follows: Linguistic Concepts, Word Structure, Sentence Structure, Oral Directions, Formulated Sentences, Recalling Sentences, Word Classes, Sentence Assembly, Semantic Relationships, Word Associations, Listening to Paragraphs. The test includes normative date for children ages 5 years, 0 months to 16 years, 11 months.

Detroit Tests of Learning Aptitude—3 (DTLA-3). (1991). Hammill, D. Austin, TX: Pro-Ed Publishers

> The test measures both general intelligence and discrete ability areas in children ages six through 17. The test includes 11 subtests: Word opposites, Design Sequences, Sentence Imitation, Reversed Letters, Story

Construction, Design Reproduction, Basic Information, Symbolic Relations, Word Sequences, Story Sequences, Picture Fragments.

Stanford-Binet Intelligence Scale, 4th edition. (1986). Thorndike, R., Hagen, E., & Sattler, J. Chicago, Il: Riverside Publishing

The test is designed to measure cognitive abilities in individuals 2 years through adult. The test assesses four cognitive areas: Verbal Reasoning, Abstract/Visual Reasoning, Quantitative Reasoning, and Short-Term Memory.

Test for Auditory Comprehension of Language—Revised (TACL-R). (1985). Carrow-Woolfolk, E. Allen, TX: DLM Teaching Resources

The test is designed to assess literal meanings of word classes, meanings of grammatical morphemes, and meanings of elaborated sentences. Norms are provided for children between the ages of 3 years, 0 months and 9 years, 11 months.

The Test of Early Language Development (TELD). (1981). Hresko, W., Reid, D., & Hammill, D. Austin, TX: Pro-Ed Publishers

The test assesses language content and form receptively and expressively. Norms are available for children 3 years, 0 months to 7 years, 11 months.

Test of Language Development—2 Primary (TOLD-2P). (1988). Newcomer, P., & Hammill, D. Austin, TX: Pro-Ed Publishers

The test assesses receptive and expressive abilities in the areas of phonology, syntax, and semantics. Norms are provided for children ages 4 years, 0 months to 8 years, 11 months. The subtests are as follows: Picture Vocabulary, Oral Vocabulary, Grammatic Understanding, Sentence Imitation, Grammatic Completion, Word Discrimination, Word Articulation.

Test of Word Finding (TWF). (1986). German, D. Allen, TX: DLM Teaching Resources

The test is designed to assess word finding skills on two dimensions: accuracy of naming and speed of naming. Norms are provided for elementary age students, 6 years, 6 months to 12 years, 11 months in grades 1 through 6. There are six sections as follows: Picture Naming: Nouns, Sentence Completion Naming; Description Naming; Picture Naming: Verbs; Picture Naming: Categories; Comprehension Assessment.

Vineland Adaptive Behavior Scales. (1984). Sparrow, S., Balla, D., & Cicchetti, D. Circle Pines, MN: American Guidance Service

The scales assess personal and social sufficiency of individuals from birth to adulthood. The instrument does not require the direct administration of tasks but instead requires a respondent who is familiar with the individual's behavior.

A P P E N D I X 3

Informal Assessment
Techniques

STORY RETELLING

METALINGUISTIC AWARENESS

COHESION

INFERENCING

PROCEDURES FOR SCORING STORY RETELLING

1. Choosing a Story

Choose a story which is clearly episodic, or, if necessary, revise an available story to increase the clarity of the episodic organization. For kindergarteners and first graders, the story should not have more than five episodes. For older children, seven or eight episode stories may be used. It is not necessary to increase the number of episodes as the child's age increases. Longer stories do not necessarily give a better picture of the child's ability to use story grammar knowledge.

To eliminate memory factors, we use picture books with the text blocked out to support the child's retelling. To eliminate the effects of complex syntax or unfamiliar vocabulary, don't be afraid to change sentence structure or vocabulary as you read the story. Just don't do anything to affect the episodic structure.

Using books with dialogue allows you to get a sense of the child's ability to put dialogue in a story. In our experience, the more familiar a child is with stories, the more likely it is that dialogue will occur. If a child is not including some dialogue in a retelling by late second grade, it is a cause for concern.

2. Preparing a Scoring Sheet

To score the child's retelling, we have found it easiest to print out the text of the story divided into episodes, with each sentence classified, down the left-hand side of a page. The child's retelling can be written in on the right hand side of the page, beside the appropriate sentence from the book. Our scoring sheet for the story *Timothy and the Night Noises*, used in Chapter 5, is shown on page 260, with one child's retelling written in, to show how this is done. (You will note that we have paraphrased the text of the story, to save space.)

3. Reading and Retelling the Story

It is essential to do this in a quiet place. You will need a tape recorder, and since you'll be transcribing the tape later, the quieter the environment the easier your task will be. First, read the story to the child, looking at the pictures together and allowing the child to make any comments he or she wishes. At the conclusion of the story reading, hand the child the book with the text blocked out, and say, "Now I'd like you to tell that story for my tape recorder." If necessary, help the child find the first page of the story, and use neutral prompts, such as "How does the story start?" or "What happened first?' Avoid focusing the child on the picture by saying "What's happening in this picture?" or "What's happening here?" The pictures are there as memory prompts for the text, and we don't want picture descriptions (although some children will give these anyway.) Language impaired children may be slow to start the retelling, and may require several prompts and many reassurances, and may also need prompts to turn the page. We have never met a child who refused to retell the story, or who expressed reluctance about talking for the tape recorder. We have, in some instances, allowed a child to say things not connected with the story, which we taped and played back so the child could hear how it would sound, before beginning the retelling.

4. Transcribing the Retelling

Transcribe the child's utterances directly onto the scoring sheet. You will need to be careful about giving the child undue credit. For example, if a child includes a particular story element out of order, put it in at the point where the child said it, and do not give the child credit for it later on in the story where it should have occurred.

We do not include prompts on our transcriptions. If you are interested in how many prompts were required for a child to get the story out, these may be indicated by putting *P* or *Prompt* in on the transcription.

5. Scoring the Child's Retelling

It is simple to identify complete episodes on the scoring sheet. The child must have one piece of the initiating event, one piece of the attempt, and one piece of the consequence for EACH episode to receive credit for that episode. You may not combine elements from different episodes to make up a whole. It is also easy to see whether there is a pattern to what the child puts in or leaves out of episodes.

Scoring Story Retelling

TIMOTHY AND THE NIGHT NOISES by Jeffrey Dinardo. Simon & Schuster, 1986

Child's Name _____

STORY GRAMMAR COMPONENTS
Setting (S)
Initiating Event (IE)
Attempt (A)
Consequence (C)
Internal Response (IR)
Ending (E)

Episodes- - Each is worth 1 point- -Total Possible = 5
If a child combines an IE with its corresponding A and C, every such combination
is called an EPISODE, and is worth 1 point .

SETTING

It was late (or bedtime) S

Timothy, Martin, Mama   S *Mommy and Timmy.*

Martin put on his pajamas   S *He's putting on his shirt.*

He hopped into bed   S

Timothy had trouble   S *and he's having problems. Mom*

Mama tucked them in S *went to help him.*

She kissed them goodnight   S

Timothy said, "I'm scared." S *He was frightened.*

"Can you leave the light on"   S

Mama said he's a big boy   S
    (frog) now

There's nothing to be afraid   S
    of

Martin is here S

Martin rolled over   S

Mama turned off the light S *and she turned off the light.*

She left the room S   *She shut the door.*

"Will you really protect me"   S

"Don't be a fathead "   S

EPISODE 1   *OK*

But then Timothy heard a noise IE   *He heard a noise.*

WOOOOOOOOO   IE

Mama help me   A

Mama came in   A   *Mom came and got him.*

"I heard a ghost"   A   *He thought it was a ghost.*

Martin made a face
    and rolled over   C

"It was only the wind"   C   *That was the wind.*

Martin rolled his eyes   C

Mama tucked him in   C

Mama sat for awhile   C   *Mom read a book to him.*

Timothy tried to sleep   C

Timothy closed his eyes   C

EPISODE 2   *No*

He heard a noise   IE   *And he heard another noise.*

CREAK   IE

He jumped into mama's lap   A   *And he jumped in his mom's
          lap.*

"What's that"   A

"It's only the chair"   C

Timothy rocked the chair   C

He went back to bed   C

EPISODE 3   *No*

He saw something moving   IE   *And he saw a shadow on the wall.*

"It's a monster"   A

"No, it's only the shadow of a tree"   C   *And mom said it was a tree outside*

Timothy felt better   IR

Mama tucked him in   C   *and she tucked him in again*

Mama left the room   C

EPISODE 4 *No*

Martin said " You're such a baby"   IE   *His brother called him a name.*

"I am not"   A

Martin made a face and rolled over   C

EPISODE 5 *OK*

Martin felt something
    tap him on the
    shoulder   IE

BOOOO   IE   *Then he went BOOO.*

Martin said "AHHH, a
    ghost   A

He ran out of the
    room   A   *He ran to mom.*

He returned with
    mama   C

Mama said there's no
    ghost   C   *There's nothing on there*

She tucked Martin in   C

She looked at Timothy   C

ENDING
Timothy is asleep   E   *He went back to sleep.*

He smiles at her   E
SHHHH   E   *He went Shhh.*

ASSESSING METALINGUISTIC AWARENESS

(These procedures are adapted from those of Kamhi and Catts [1986].)

1. Sentence Division

This task provides a measure of word or lexical awareness.

Instructions: You're going to hear some sentences. After each sentence, I will stop the tape and ask you to say the whole sentence back to me. Then I will ask you to say a little bit of the sentence. I will keep asking you to say a little bit until you can't make it any smaller. Let me give you an example. I will say a sentence. Ready? *Jack and Jill went up the hill.* Now I will say a little bit of that sentence. *Jack and Jill.* That was a little bit of the sentence. Now I will say a little bit of Jack and Jill. Ready? *Jack.* That was a little bit of Jack and Jill. Do you understand what we're doing? Let's try one. I'll say a sentence, and see if you can say a little bit of it. *Babies don't cry.* Now you say the whole sentence back to me. Now can you say a little bit of that? If the child responds with *babies*, then ask for another little bit. If the child says *don't cry*, repeat the phrase and ask for a little bit of *don't cry*. Continue until the child has reached the level of individual words, or until the child cannot continue. Give corrective feedback if necessary. (The child is asked to repeat the whole sentence to make sure it can be held in working memory. The goal here is to find out whether the child can segment the sentence to the level of individual words. If the child seems not to understand, move to a two-word sentence, and give a few more practice items. Give four examples, providing corrective feedback if necessary, and proceed with the task. The child should be encouraged to divide each multiword phrase into separate words before attempting to divide the remainder of the sentence. If the child's initial response to *tell me a little bit* is an individual word, continue to ask for a little bit until all the words of the sentence have been given.)

Scoring: Give one point for each division the child is able to make. The total number of points for each sentence is equal to the number of words in the sentence minus one. A five word sentence, for example, could be divided four times.

Testing Items

1. Daddy fell.	6. The baby was happy.
2. Mommy ran home.	7. We saw the big tree.
3. The cat left.	8. The man came to my house.

    4. The dog ran away.   9. Mommy put the ball in the box.
    5. Daddy made the boat.   10. The boy broke his new bike

2. Word Division

This task provides a measure of phonological awareness.

Bisyllabic Words

Instructions: Now we're going to do the same thing with some words. We will hear a word, and I will ask you to say a little bit of it. Let me give you an example. Here's a word. Ready? *Monday.* Now I will say a little bit of it. Ready? *Mon.* Mon is a little bit of Monday. Now you try one. Ready? *Baby.* (Your goal with bisyllabic words is to get to the level of the syllable. Give example items until the child seems to understand the task. If the child misses three in a row, stop the task.)

Scoring: Give one point for each word if the child responds with one of the syllables. Give no points if the child responds in any other way.

    Testing Items—Bisyllabic

1. airplane	5. monkey	9. beside
2. football	6. pencil	10. penny
3. pancake	7. window	
4. doctor	8. open	

Monosyllabic Words

Instructions: Now we're going to hear some other words. I will ask you to tell me a little bit of the word again. First I'll do one. Ready? *Man.* Now I'll say a little bit of "man." Ready? *an.* "An" is a little bit of "man." Now you try one. Ready? *Bat.* Say a little bit of "bat." (Your goal here is to get to a level smaller than the whole word. It is not necessary to get to the individual phoneme level. Give four examples, providing corrective feedback if necessary, and proceed with the testing items. If the child misses three items in a row, stop and proceed to the next task.)

Scoring: Give one point for each word if the child can give some part of it other than the entire word. Give no points if the child gives back the whole word, or gives a sound not a part of the word.

    Testing items—Monosyllabic

1. plane	5. doc	9. late
2. foot	6. key	10. meet

3. hot	7. pen
4. cake	8. deep

3. Elision

This task provides a measure of phonological awareness by evaluating knowledge of phonemic segments

Instructions: I'm going to say a word to you. You say the word just like I do. Then I'm going to tell you a part to leave off, either at the beginning or the end of the word. You say the word, leaving off the part I tell you to. I'll try one first, to give you an example. Ready? Say the word *cow*. "COW." See, I said it exactly the same way. Now the next part. Ready? *Say the word cow without the /k/ sound. "ow"* See, I took off the sound /k/, and I got "ow." Now you try one. Say the word *man*. Now say the word without the /m/ sound. (When asking the child to omit a sound, do not give the letter name. Give the sound made by the letter. Give three examples, providing corrective feedback. If the child misses three items in a row, stop the task.)

Scoring: Give one point if the child's response is correct, give no points if it is incorrect.

Testing Items—Elision: the sound to be eliminated is in parentheses.

1. (t)old	7. (b)ring	13. far(m)
2. (b)lend	8. (s)pin	14. car(d)
3. (t)all	9. sun(k)	15. for(k)
4. (n)ice	10. bus(t)	16. star(t)
5. (s)top	11. pin(k)	
6. (n)ear	12. ben(t)	

4. Morpheme Judgment

This task provides a measure of a child's ability to access morphological information

Instructions: I have a puppet here who can't talk well. I want you to help him talk. He is going to say a sentence, and I want you to tell him whether the sentence is a good one. If it's not a good one, I want you to make it better. Give the following three examples: *He is eating cake. Tomorrow he go school. Brush your teeth.* After each example sentence, ask the child whether the sentence is good or bad. If the child says it is bad, ask for a good version. After giving the examples, and providing corrective feedback, proceed with the testing items.

Scoring: Give one point if the child makes a correct judgment about the sentence. Give another point if the child can correct the incorrect sentence.

Testing Items—Morpheme Judgment

1. Steven dog was lost.
2. I tried get the book.
3. Nancy is smaller than Karen.
4. He already eaten dinner.
5. Yesterday he see a movie.
6. Kathy has three dogs.
7. John is big than Dave.
8. She needs to get home.
9. He not want to play today.
10. She walked quiet into the room.
11. They throwing the stick.
12. Where the coat is?
13. Yesterday he ran to school.
14. John has two book.
15. Usually they walks to school.
16. The girl painted picture.

ASSESSING KNOWLEDGE OF COHESION

Children's story and textbooks are good sources for text to use for checking a child's comprehension of cohesion. It will be important to use text that is suitable to the level of the child being tested. In general, we don't check for knowledge of cohesion before second grade, both because children tend not to use many cohesive devices themselves until second grade, and also because many language impaired children have difficulty simply recalling enough of the text to answer the questions unless they can follow along as you read. This should not be regarded as a memory test. The child can look at the text as you ask questions. If the child does not understand cohesion, looking at the text won't be a help.

1. Text at a Second Grade Level

Read the text to the child, allowing the child to follow along.

Mary Jones and her mother were busy getting ready for Valentine's Day. Mary was busy cutting out valentines for her friends at school. Her brother Tommy was watching her work. Her mother was busy in the bedroom. She was making a dress for Mary for a party. Soon a neighbor came to the door. "Come in," said Mary to Mrs. King. "See my valentines." Mrs. King said, "I have been making valentines too. But I put my valentines in the oven to bake. Would you children like some of them?" Mary and Tommy each ate a cookie.

Instructions—Now I'm going to say some things about what we just read. If what I say is true, you say "yes." If what I say is not true, you say "no." Ready? (Allow the child to look at the questions as you read them.)

1. Mary's mother was busy. *(yes)*
2. Mary was cutting out valentines for her mother's friends. *(no)*
3. Tommy was watching his mother work. *(no)*
4. The neighbor's name was Mrs. King. *(yes)*
5. Mrs. King's valentines were cookies. *(yes)*

2. Text at a Third/Fourth Grade Level

We adapted text from the book *Blaze and the Forest Fire* by C. W. Anderson (1966) for the assessment presented here.

Read the text to the child, allowing the child to follow along.

Billy was a boy who loved horses more than anything else in the world. He loved his own pony, Blaze, best of all. After his father and mother gave him Blaze, Billy spent most of his time with the pony. Blaze would come whenever Billy called. He seemed to like the rides through the woods or along the roads as much as Billy did. Billy felt sure that Blaze understood him when he talked; and the pony really did seem to understand what Billy said. Billy's dog, Rex, usually went with them on their rides. But one day he was sick; so Billy's mother kept him at home. It was a beautiful day, and Billy decided to ride along a little winding road. It passed through some woods, and not many people used it. Both Billy and Blaze liked to ride through the woods, because there were so many things to see. They always met rabbits and squirrels and saw many birds.

Instructions—Now I'm going to say some things about what we just read. If what I say is true, you say "yes." If what I say is not true, you say "no." Ready? (Allow the child to look at the questions as you read them.)

1. Billy's horse was named Blaze. *(yes)*
2. Billy's father and mother gave him Blaze. (yes)
3. Billy spent most of his time with his father and mother. *(no)*
4. Billy liked rides through the woods or along the roads. *(yes)*
5. Billy understood Blaze when he talked. *(no)*
6. Billy talked to his pony. *(yes)*
7. Billy's dog was named Rex. *(yes)*
8. Billy was sick one day. *(no)*
9. Not many people rode along the little winding road. *(yes)*
10. Blaze saw rabbits and squirrels. *(yes)*

3. Text at a Fifth/Sixth Grade Level

We adapted this text from a sixth grade Social Studies book, *People in Time and Place: Western Hemisphere*, published by Silver, Burdett, & Ginn, 1991.

At the time Christopher Columbus made his famous voyages, people in Europe believed that all the major land areas in the world had already been discovered. Many people thought that Asia and the surrounding islands were much closer to Europe than they really are. They were unaware that if they sailed west, they would find two huge continents between Europe and Asia. They were also unaware of the existence of the vast Pacific Ocean.

The discoveries of Columbus and other daring explorers surprised Europeans. They thought the new lands could be nothing more than islands near Asia in the Atlantic Ocean. Little by little, as more explorers tried to sail around these supposed islands, the true shape and size of the New World became apparent.

Instructions: I'm going to say some things about the text we just read. If what I say is true, you say "yes." If what I say is not true, you say "no." (Allow the child to read the questions along with you.)

1. People in Europe once thought that Asia was closer to Europe than it really is. *(yes)*
2. People in Europe thought that if they sailed west they would find Europe and Asia. *(no)*
3. People in Asia were unaware of the existence of the Pacific Ocean. *(no)*
4. The new lands discovered by Columbus were continents. *(yes)*
5. Europeans were surprised to discover explorers. *(no)*
6. The explorers thought the new lands were islands near Asia. *(no)*
7. The continents discovered by Columbus and other explorers were between Asia and Europe. *(yes)*
8. The size of the New World became apparent only after explorers tried to sail around it. *(yes)*
9. The size of the New World was discovered quite suddenly. *(no)*
10. The explorers knew the true shape of the New World from the beginning. *(no)*

ASSESSING INFERENCING ABILITIES

We have unashamedly lifted the procedures for assessing interferencing from Bishop and Adams (1992). The only changes we have made involved changing some British English to American English. The subjects in the Bishop and Adams study were between the ages of 8 and 12 years, so the items should be useful for children in that age group.

Instructions: I'm going to tell you some short stories, and after each story, I will ask you some questions. You need to listen carefully to the stories so you will be able to answer the questions.

Story #1

Jane looked in her piggy bank and found that she had three dollars. She set off down the road past the grocery store carrying a package for her mother under her arm. When she got to the candy store, she put down the package so that she could point to the jar of green M&M's, which were her favorites. But while her back was turned a man sneaked into the store and took the package. A policewoman at the police station was very kind to Jane but she was still very upset.

Questions (Note: questions are coded *L* for literal recall, *I* for inferencing)

I. Where does Jane keep her money?
I. What did Jane take out of her piggy bank?
I. Why did she take her money out?
L. What did Jane carry under her arm?
L. Which store did she walk past?
L. Which store did she go into?
L. What did she point to in the shop?
I. Why did she point to the jar of M&M's?
L. Who took the package?
I. Who did the package belong to?
I. Why did the man take the package?
I. Where is Jane at the end of the story?
L. Who helped Jane at the end of the story?
I. Why is Jane upset at the end of the story?

Story #2

There was a huge burst of flame from the bottom of the rocket as it took off from the launching pad. The chief astronaut wore a blue spacesuit. He was sitting at the controls studying a map of the planet Mars. The navigator wore a yellow spacesuit. He was standing at the window and was excited because he could see the planet Mars. The Martians had a TV screen on which they could see outer space. They saw a spaceship on their screen. When the spaceship landed, the Martians were hiding in a crater. The spaceship took off in a hurry when the Martians started throwing rocks.

Questions (Note: questions are coded *L* for literal recall, *I* for inferencing)

L. What was taking off from the launching pad?
L. Where was the burst of flame?

I. Where was the rocket heading for when it set off from the launching pad?

L. What was the man in the blue spacesuit looking at?

I. What did the man in the yellow spacesuit see?

I. Where were the two astronauts when they saw the planet Mars?

I. How do you think the astronauts felt when they saw the planet Mars?

L. What did the Martians see on their TV screen?

I. Who was in the spaceship that the Martians saw on their TV screen?

L. Where did the Martians hide?

I. Why did the Martians hide?

L. What did the Martians do with the rocks?

I. How do you think the astronauts felt when their spaceship took off?

I. How do you think the Martians felt when the spaceship went away?

Story #3

Mike was riding his bike down the road and decided to turn in through a gate. Just behind the fence, there was a pile of stuff someone had thrown away. Right on top there was an old baby buggy. Mike ran to find his friends, who were playing in the woods. "Come and see what I've found," he said. Mike and his friends climbed to the top of the pile and got the buggy down. They took the top part off and hammered an old board into position above the base of the buggy. Mike got into the go-cart and raced down the track on it while his friends cheered.

Questions (Note: questions are coded *L* for literal recall, *I* for inferencing)

L. Where did Mike turn off the road?

L. What was on top of the pile of stuff?

I. What was the buggy doing on top of the pile?

I. What did Mike think when he first saw the buggy?

L. Who did Mike go to find?

I. Why did he tell his friends about it?

L. What did they do with the top part of the buggy?

L. What did they hammer onto the buggy?

I. Why did the children take the top of the buggy off?

I. Where did Mike get the hammer from?

L. What did Mike do when he'd finished making the go-cart?

L. What did the children do at the end of the story?

I. How did the children feel when they saw Mike racing on the go-cart?

I. What do you think Mike will do with the go-cart now?

A P P E N D I X 4

Selected Children's Literature

CHILDREN'S LITERATURE REFERRED TO IN THE TEXT

CHILDREN'S LITERATURE WE LIKE TO USE

CHILDREN'S LITERATURE REFERRED TO IN THE TEXT

Aardema, Verna (1975). *Why Mosquitos Buzz in People's Ears.* New York, NY: Dial Books for Young Readers

Dinardo, Jeffrey (1986). *Timothy and the Night Noises.* New York, NY: Simon and Schuster Publishing

Ets, Marie Hall (1978). *Gilberto and the Wind.* New York, NY: Penguin Books

Gibbons, Gail (1988). *Farming.* New York, NY: Holiday House

Gurney, Eric and Nancy (1965). *The King The Mice and The Cheese.* New York, NY: Random House, Inc.

Johnson, Crockett (1959). *Herald and the Purple Crayon.* New York, NY: Scholastic, Inc.

Keats, Ezra Jack (1976). *The Snowy Day.* New York, NY: Puffin Books

Lester, Helen (1988). *Tacky the Penguin.* New York, NY: Trumpet Club

Lester, Helen (1987). *Pookins Gets Her Way.* Boston, MA: Houghton Mifflin Co.

Lobel, Arnold (1977). *Mouse Soup.* New York, NY: Harper Trophy

Mayer, Mercer (1967). *A Boy, A Dog, and A Frog.* New York, NY: Dial Books for Young Readers

Mayer, Mercer (1992). *There's a Nightmare in My Closet.* New York, NY: Puffin Books

Siebert, Diane (1989). *Heartland.* New York, NY: Harper Trophy

Suess, Dr. (1963). *Hop On Pop.* New York, NY: Random House Inc.

Suess, Dr. (1957). *The Cat in the Hat.* New York, NY: Random House Inc

Viorst, Judith (1972). *Alexander and the Terrible, Horrible, No Good, Very Bad Day.* New York, NY: Aladdin Books; MacMillan Publishing Co.

White, E.B. (1952). *Charlotte's Web.* New York, NY: Harper Collins

Ziefert, Harriet (1987). *Jason's Bus Ride.* New York, NY: Puffin Books

CHILDREN'S LITERATURE WE LIKE TO USE
(Arranged by Category)

Episodic Structure

Bourgeois, P. and Clark, B. (1986). *Franklin in the Dark.* New York, NY: Scholastic.

Anderson, C.W. (1938). *Blaze and the Forest Fire.* New York, NY: Aladdin Books, MacMillan Publishing Co.

Hogrogian, Nonny (1971). *One Fine Day*. New York, NY: The Trumpet Club

McPhail, David (1972). *The Bear's Toothache*. Boston, MA: Little, Brown and Co.

Munsch, Robert (1985). *Thomas' Snowsuit*. Toronto, Canada: Annick Press Ltd.

Roy, Ron (1979). *Three Ducks Went Wandering*. New York, NY: Scholastic

Rey, Margret and H.A. *The Curious George Collection*. Boston, MA: Houghton Mifflin Co.

Predictable Books

Campbell, Rod (1982). *Dear Zoo*. New York, NY: The Trumpet Club

Carle, Eric (1987). *Have You Seen My Cat?* New York, NY: Scholastic.

Shaw, Charles (1947). *It Looked Like Spilt Milk*. New York, NY: Scholastic

Williams, Sue (1989). *I Went Walking*. New York, NY: Harcourt Brace Jovanovich, Publishers

Ziefert, Harriet (1988). *Here Comes A Bus*. New York, NY: Puffin Books

Wordless Books

Carle, Eric (1971). *Do You Want To Be My Friend?* New York, NY: Harper Trophy

DePaola, Tomie (1978). *Pancakes for Breakfast*. New York, NY: Harcourt Brace Jovanovich Publishers

Turk, Hanne (1983). *Raking Leaves With Max*. Natick, MA: Alphabet Press

Turkle, Brinton (1976). *Deep In The Forest*. New York, NY: The Trumpet Club

Main Idea and Inferencing/Predicting

Cameron, Ann. *The Julian Series*. New York, NY: Bullseye Books

Chardiet, Bernice (1994). *Something Is Coming*. New York, NY: Puffin Books

Chardiet, B. and Maccarone, G. *The School Friends Series*. New York, NY: Scholastic

Guarino, Deborah (1989). *Is Your Mama a Llama?* New York, NY: Scholastic

Kellogg, Steven (1971). *Can I Keep Him?* New York, NY: Penguin Books
Oppenheim, Joanne (1992). *The Show-And-Tell Frog.* New York, NY: Bantam Books
Sharmot, Margorie. *Nate the Great Series.* New York, NY: Dell Publishing
Steptoe, John (1984). *The Story of Jumping Mouse.* New York, NY: Scholastic

Metalinguistics/Phonological Awareness

Kalish, Muriel and Lionel (1993). *Bears On The Stairs.* New York, NY: Scholastic
Martin, Bill Jr. and Archambault, John (1989). *Chicka Chicka Boom Boom.* New York, NY: Scholastic
McMillan, Bruce (1990). *One Sun.* New York, NY: Scholastic
Patz, Nancy (1983). *Moses Supposes His Toeses Are Roses.* New York, NY: Harcourt Brace Jovanovich Publishers

Scripting

Barton, Byron (1982). *Airport.* New York, NY: Thomas Y. Crowell
Carlson, Nancy (1982). *Harriet's Recital.* New York, NY: Puffin Books
Winthrop, ELizabeth (1989). *Sledding.* New York, NY: Harper Collins

I N D E X

American Speech-Language-Hearing
 Association (ASHA)
 specific language impairment
  definition, 11–12
Assessment. *See also* Testing; Tests
 child identified after starting
  school, 31–34
 classroom based model, 43–54
 clinical approach, 14–16
 collaborative model, 43–54
 conversational
  analysis, 75–89
  sample
   analysis, 89
   gathering, 88–89
 informal techniques, 258–270
  cohesion, 266–268
  inferencing, 268–270
  metalinguistic awareness
   morpheme judgment, 265
   sentence division, 259–263
   word division, 263–265
  story retelling scoring, 258–259
 preschool child in school setting,
  24–27
 scripted event recounting, 121–123
 standard deviation defined, 6
 story frameworks, 130–133
 strategies, 1–35

test scores and language impairment
 determination, 4, 6–14

Brainstorming, clinical
 child identified after starting
  school, 30–31, 54–57
 intervention, 54–57, 59–61
 preschool child in school setting,
  21–24, 59–61

Case histories
 child identified after starting
  school, 28–34
 cohesion, 181–192
 main idea identification, 192–199
 metalinguistic awareness, 178–181
 phonological awareness, 178–181
 preschool child in school setting,
  19–27
 scripts, 139–144
 stories (schemata), 139–143,
  147–154
Chapter I federal program, 22,
 179–180
Classroom based intervention. *See*
 under Intervention

275